THE PRACTICE MANAGER LIBRARY

Premises and Information Technology
your questions answered

Lyn Longridge

RADCLIFFE MEDICAL PRESS

Radcliffe Medical Press Ltd
18 Marcham Road, Abingdon, Oxon OX14 1AA

British Library Cataloguing in Publication Data

A catalogue record for this book is available from the British Library

ISBN 1 85775 254 6

Library of Congress Cataloguing-in-Publication Data is available.

Typeset by Acorn Bookwork, Salisbury, Wiltshire
Printed and bound by Biddles Ltd, Guildford and King's Lynn

Contents

About the author

Lyn Longridge has worked in general practice since the 1980s, starting her career in Devon and moving subsequently to Tewkesbury. In 1993, she began writing articles on practice management for specialist journals and in 1996 she was invited to serve on the editorial board of *Practice Manager*. Lyn is a member of the General Practitioner Writers Association, a society that promotes the work of their members, mostly GPs, on all subjects. She is the author of *Managing and Communicating* and *Finance and Administration*, the first two books in The Practice Manager Library series.

Lyn is currently a freelance management consultant troubleshooting in practices that are struggling to cope with constant change. She also trains GPs and their practice managers in the use of the Maclean McNicoll GP accounts software. She organizes occasional training courses for practice managers under the auspices of the West Oxfordshire College at Witney and for the Dorset Health Authority.

Acknowledgements

I should like to acknowledge the help I have received from several people during the preparation of this book. Guy Bridgewater, technical director of PCTI (Professional Computer Training and Installation) read a first draft of the section on information technology and helped greatly by supplying up-to-date technical information and his vision of the future of IT in general practice. Drs Andy Rigby and Chris Mimnagh, GPs with a particular enthusiasm and expertise in computing and its application to general practice, kindly spared the time to offer me the GP's view of the likely future applications for practice computer systems. Pat Moreton, manager of the Holts Medical Centre at Newent kindly read the first draft of this book and made some useful comments on premises issues.

As usual, my son Edward has kept me supplied with information on possible future developments in primary care gained during the day-to-day management of a practice in Dorset. His comments on some of the aspects of practice management covered in this book have been particularly helpful.

I should like to thank my editor at Radcliffe Medical Press, Jamie Etherington, for his help and patience in guiding me through the production of this and previous books in The Practice Manager Library series.

Finally, my thanks to all those unsung practice managers whom I have met during the past year in practices up and down the country and whose views and concerns have influenced my choice of subjects chosen for inclusion in this book.

Lyn Longridge
May 1998

For Alison

Introduction

This book is the third in The Practice Manager Library series. The first explored the management and communication skills necessary to run a busy practice and also identified some of the professionals who now constitute the primary health care team. The second covered issues relating to the finance and administration of the practice. This third book will concentrate on matters relating to the management of premises and information technology in general practice.

Most practices are facing the need to expand their premises as more and more services are devolved to primary care. Many inner-city practices, often run by a GP single-handedly are located in cramped, unsuitable buildings. These doctors see little hope of obtaining funds from hard-pressed health authorities in order to pay for much-needed expansion and refurbishment of their practices. This book addresses possible alternative sources of funding for such developments and also identifies other ways of relieving the pressure on premises by setting up satellite or branch surgeries.

Most practices are now computerized although there are some

still unwilling to switch to modern technology, abandoning their tried and tested manual systems. However, the degree to which individual practices make use of this technology varies tremendously, often depending on whether there is a partner or manager within the practice who has a particular interest in computers. So often the expensive equipment is used merely for repeat prescriptions and patient registration when it could be used in so many different ways to facilitate better management of the practice. Ways of using computers and allied peripherals to better effect are explored in the second half of the book.

The present government seems keen to retain the benefits of fundholding, one of which they identify in the White Paper published in December 1997 as the management expertise that general practices have gained in obtaining health care for their patients. In fact, they state that it is 'the management expertise of GPs' but I rather suspect that many practices would agree that any management expertise lies with the practice manager and/or fund manager. The government is keen to harness this expertise but anxious to lose the perceived disadvantages of the fundholding system such as the increase in bureaucracy and high management costs involved. Perhaps by adapting premises and utilizing information technology, practices will be able to provide a more cost-effective health care service for patients in their own community.

In the following pages I hope to address some of the problems GPs might encounter in adapting their practices to the ever-increasing needs and demands of patients in the primary care sector.

Lyn Longridge
May 1998

In the interests of clarity, throughout the book it has been assumed that all practice managers are female and all GPs male, although this is clearly not the case in most practices.

1

Premises

Practices throughout the country are housed in premises in a variety of styles and sizes. Some are fortunate to have space on the ground floor to house all the consulting rooms and offices, while others have to use upper storeys in order to provide the services required. Inner-city and town premises are likely to be more constrained by cramped premises than those in rural areas. However, rural practices are increasingly providing more and more services such as chiropody and physiotherapy within the practice, saving patients the journey to the nearest hospital.

The increase in demand for complementary therapies has meant that practitioners of osteopathy, acupuncture and homoeopathy are frequently to be found offering their services at the surgery also. All this combined with the increased patient expectation for health care generally is putting tremendous pressure on practices to expand.

It is usually the practice manager's job to look after the practice premises, ensuring that they are well maintained and cleaned to a high standard as befits a centre providing health care services. In the following section, ways of providing additional space in which to offer such services are explored and ways of funding such expansion will be discussed. Advice on many aspects regarding insuring, valuing, securing and maintaining the building will be covered.

▲ Question 1: Extending premises

Our surgery is very cramped at present and we are hoping to introduce clinics by complementary therapists soon, although there is nowhere to put them. The partners are very keen to stay put in our present premises but there doesn't seem to be much room to expand. What can we do to make more space available?

You should first check that you have considered all the alternatives such as rescheduling some of the existing surgeries and clinics so that, if necessary, the same consulting room can be used by a series of practitioners in rotation – the system known as 'Box and Cox'. GPs are often reluctant to allow others to use their consulting rooms because they dislike the inevitable upheaval and misplacing of various pieces of equipment. However, to obtain optimum use of the present premises serial occupancy is certainly an option worth exploring.

You will probably already have moved most of the administrative staff to offices on upper floors if there are any. This releases more accessible space for patient contact and is an obvious first step to take when trying to release more ground floor accommodation for consulting. Some of the consulting rooms can, of course, be on the first or second floors if there is a lift available for disabled patients or if a treatment room is easily accessible on the ground floor in which any patients unable to cope with stairs can be seen by their GP. Medical records can be stored on an upper floor also, with the proviso that there is an efficient lift or dumbwaiter system for moving notes around.

However, you may have already considered all the above possible solutions to pressure for ground floor space and may still be left with cramped premises. What are the possibilities for expansion? Are there adjacent properties which might be coming up for sale in the near future? Is there a property nearby – but not necessarily next door – which the practice could acquire and perhaps put the secretariat or one or two consulting rooms in, with the necessary computer and telephone links to the main building?

If all the above prove impracticable, you will then be left with no alternative but to improve the layout of the present premises in order to gain more space. Have you any garden you can build into? Can you build upwards? Can you reallocate the space within the building, perhaps getting rid of unnecessary corridors or surplus storage areas to improve availability of rooms?

A good architect who has experience of GP surgery projects is essential. He will need a clear idea of just what additional space the GPs hope to gain and how much they can afford to spend on acquiring it. It will be his task to investigate any potential problems regarding planning permission and advise you accordingly.

At all stages it is obviously vital to keep both staff and patients informed of any imminent changes to the layout of the building. Staff can become quite territorial about their own working space and it is important to involve them in any discussions about possible moves.

Any surveyor or solicitor whom you consult about the building should also know something about general practice and the way GPs are funded and how their income is derived.

▲ Question 2: Green-field site

Our premises no longer provide sufficient accommodation for the needs of our expanding practice. We are considering the possibility of building new premises from scratch in a location not far from our present surgery. Where or how do we start?

You should first decide whether a new building is the best possible option. Have you considered extending your present premises? How about a branch surgery? Would that help to reduce the pressure on the main surgery? Is your list likely to increase further in future or might it begin to wither?

If you have decided that a new building is the only feasible option, your first step should be to start discussions with the cost rent officer at the health authority. Do they have any funds available for cost rent in the immediate future? What is the timescale likely to be if you do decide to go ahead and build? Finding a suitable site on which to build at a price that the practice can afford can often prove to be a stumbling block. Have you made enquiries locally or perhaps the partners have a possible site in mind? GPs are often well placed to learn of likely sites that might be coming up for sale.

You will obviously have to look at some of the various ways of financing the building. Are the partners willing to take out a loan? Do they already have a mortgage on their present premises? Will the same lender consider making them a further loan? Banks and building societies are not always conversant with the cost rent scheme. You will need to explain that cost rental payments from the health authority are guaranteed and, having given these assurances to the lender, the partners should be able to obtain a favourable interest rate.

If it proves difficult to raise the necessary funds, you might want to consider alternatives. Do the partners actually want to own the building or might they prefer to find a developer who would be willing to build the new surgery and then lease it back to the practice? This takes away the worry of funding the project but the downside is that it means that the partners lose any opportunity to gain from capital appreciation.

Have you considered the Private Finance Initiative (PFI)? Under the PFI, capital projects are funded in partnership with the private sector. The private sector company will make its profit from lease or rental income. In some areas the health authority, social services and private finance have jointly funded the building of a large primary care centre.

Once you have taken all the above into consideration and the partners have made their decision, you should warn them that the whole project is likely to take far longer than is at first envisaged. However good the initial planning, it will almost certainly be fraught with unexpected problems, so be prepared to devote a great deal of time over the coming months to planning and negotiating.

▲ Question 3: Branch surgeries

We have three branch surgeries attached to this practice. It is a nightmare of logistics trying to ensure that staff are available to cover and a GP to attend each of the surgeries. What might be the implications if we were to close one or more of them?

You need to ask yourself some searching questions before embarking on any course of action with regard to the closure of a branch surgery.

- Do you want to retain all your present patients?
- Are some of them only registered with your practice because of the convenience of a branch surgery near their homes?
- Might they register with another practice if the branch surgery were to be closed?
- Do you keep the branch surgeries open longer than is strictly necessary?
- Could you manage with fewer surgeries held at the various branches?
- Do you need any staff at all at the smaller surgeries that are only open once or twice a week?
- Could the GP manage on his own, taking notes from the main surgery as required or accessing patient notes on the computer via a landline?
- Would open surgeries rather than booked appointments be more practical?

If you feel that there would not be a large drifting away of patients if you were to close one or more of the branches, then I would suggest it is probably time you looked into the possibility. You must be aware of the rules regarding dispensing to patients. There is always the danger that if you close a branch, you might lose patients and this in turn might mean that 20% of the practice's patients no longer live more than one mile distant from the nearest pharmacy. The partnership would therefore no longer fulfil the eligibility requirements for dispensing. It might also mean that you lose patients for whom you are currently claiming rural practice payments.

▲ Question 4: Professionals – architects, surveyors, lawyers

We are in the process of planning an extension to our practice premises. How do we go about choosing a suitable architect?

The first pitfall to avoid is allowing the doctors to choose as architect, a golfing buddy of the senior partner or, worse still, perhaps a patient of one of the GPs. This is seldom a good basis on which to make such an important choice and if the chosen professional is particularly friendly with one of the doctors, this can lead to decisions being made without due consultation with the whole partnership. This can prove to be very divisive and may put the whole project at risk.

The ideal architect will be one who is well versed in the idiosyncrasies of general practice and its requirements. Your health authority should be able to provide you with a list of architects who have worked on other GP premises projects locally. They will not, however, be able or willing to recommend a particular firm. It is important to contact the individual practices who have had work done and ask them for a reference. Their opinion is likely to be particularly helpful and any comments, especially those made informally on the telephone, can be very revealing. One practice approached in this way said that their architect had produced some wonderful plans for their new extension, but these did not take into account the workings of a busy practice. Waiting areas were too small, there was no privacy for callers at the reception desk and the personal security of members of staff was not taken into account in the planning, despite the fact that all these issues had been raised in preliminary discussions. You should plan to visit one or two of the practices for which the architects have worked and look at the completed building. Is this the kind of design you might be seeking for your premises?

By speaking to all the practices concerned you should be able to build up a picture of which firm is likely to produce the kind of plans that would suit your practice. It is not usual to approach more than one and ask for draft ideas for an extension, although in special circumstances this has been done. If the firm wants the commission badly enough, they might be prepared to speculate a little of their time in producing rough sketches of their ideas. However, normally you make your choice following recommendation by previous GP clients and visits to their premises and then have an initial meeting with the chosen architect to thrash out ideas.

It is important to ensure that the architect is aware from the beginning of the total budget available for the project and it should be stressed that this must not be exceeded. It is certainly a good idea to have a contingency fund into which you can dip if costs do begin to escalate and the budget is breached. Again, do not forget to keep the health authority informed at every stage of your deliberations. You will need to obtain written confirmation of the availability of cost rent on the proposed project before making any firm commitments to invest in new premises (*see* Question **20**).

▲ Question 5: Surgeries within superstores

I work part time managing the practice of a single-handed GP. He has recently been approached by a supermarket chain and asked if he would be interested in moving into premises adjoining a new superstore which they are planning to build in our practice area. What points should he consider when making his decision?

There are several practices already housed in premises owned by large superstores. Often there is also a pharmacy adjoining the proposed GP surgery. The main advantage to the GP is that he will have premises of a standard which, had he had to fund them himself, would probably have been way beyond his reach. The supermarket chain gains because they believe that the presence of a GP 'adds value', attracting potential customers to the store's own products and its in-house pharmacy.

It is vital that an architect experienced in the planning of GP premises is brought in at an early stage of negotiations. It is also important that additional space is made available to allow for the inevitable expansion of the practice in years to come. With the shift from secondary to primary care, more and more services are being provided within general practice and it is likely that this trend will continue. Also, it is possible that more patients will want to register with the practice given the convenience of the location for many of the supermarket customers. The GP should consider whether he might be willing to take on a partner or employ an assistant, if this expansion in his list were to take place.

The management team of the supermarket chain are likely to be experts at negotiating and so it is important to make sure that the terms agreed for the concession are not unreasonable. The negotiators will need to be made aware of how a GP is paid (quarterly in arrears) and to take this into account when negotiating appropriate rental payments.

▲ Question 6: Pharmacies within practices/practices within pharmacies

I have heard of practices that have let space in their premises to an independent pharmacist but recently someone mentioned a large pharmacy that is leasing a room within their store for the use of GPs. What do you think of this idea?

There are indeed practices which have let space within their practice for a pharmacy. This can work to the advantage of both parties. However, there has been some discussion about the possibility of pharmacy chains employing GPs directly, reversing the situation. Most doctors working in general practice do not consider this an ideal solution as they value their independent contractor status too much to risk losing their autonomy by being employees of a commercial concern. Pharmacy chains are keen that the expertise of their highly trained pharmacists should be better utilized and having a GP with whom they liaise closely is one way of facilitating this.

Boots the Chemist plan to offer space in up to six of their larger stores during 1998. They will be inviting Sinclair Montrose to take on the lease as part of a two-year trial. Sinclair Montrose will then rent the premises to NHS GPs who will be expected to share the site with private doctors, providing a walk-in primary care service. All support services, including receptionists and nurses, will be organized, employed and provided by the company. The NHS GPs will be expected to buy the services of the nurses and receptionists.

The idea is that such surgeries will be in high street sites in market towns and Boots claim to be attempting to regenerate the high street by the introduction of this idea. The GPs would continue practising from their main surgery premises but would have a branch centrally on the high street within the pharmacy which might prove to be a more convenient location for some of the patients to visit. (However, *see* Question **3** for some of the possible drawbacks of having a branch surgery.)

There was some concern expressed that patients might feel they had to take their prescriptions to the pharmacist working from the same premises as their GP rather than to any other. However, GPs are not permitted to refer patients to a specific pharmacy and no pressure could or should be brought to bear on patients to do this. However, if the pharmacy is in close proximity to the practice, patients will probably welcome the opportunity to consult the pharmacist on minor medical matters in the absence of the GP and are also likely to take their prescriptions to be made up.

▲ Question 7: One-stop health shop

I read somewhere about a new one-stop health shop. Can you tell me what this might include and whether this is likely to be the way forward for primary care?

Perhaps you are thinking about the Fountain Medical Centre in Leeds which opened in 1997 and provides space for outpatient clinics, minor surgery, an X-ray department and an endoscopy unit, together with accommodation leased to a pharmacist, dentist and optician. Various other therapies are also available at the centre including chiropractic, physiotherapy, podiatry, chiropody, hypnotherapy, homoeopathy, remedial massage, aromatherapy, reflexology, counselling and acupuncture. Patients are referred to some of these practitioners who are paid out of the fundholding budget; others treat patients on a private basis and the patients are billed directly by the practitioner.

Consultants employed by the local trust hold surgical and ophthalmology outpatient clinics at the centre and patients from other practices can also attend these sessions. The ophthalmology outpatients are seen within the optician's premises because of the

specialized equipment available there. Outreach clinics in gynaecology and audiology are also available but only for patients registered with the practice.

The centre has its own X-ray facilities and is considering the
introduction of an ultrasound service. As an accredited provider of
endoscopies, the practice has a contract with the health authority
as well as with local fundholding practices and can thus offer the
service to patients belonging to any practice in the area. There is
also a sizeable seminar room available which is used mainly for
staff training and PGEA meetings.

There are other practices in the North such as one at Wakefield
and another near Halifax which are developing centres along
similar lines but, unlike the Fountain Medical Centre, these are
developer-led projects. A developer acquires the site and builds all
the facilities which he then leases to the various practitioners. The
GPs do not have the problem of obtaining funding for the project
but on the other hand, nor do they have the opportunity to benefit
from possible capital appreciation or the increasing rents charge-
able to tenants.

It is likely that the government will continue to encourage the
shift of focus from secondary to primary care and so other
practices will almost certainly follow the lead of the Fountain
Medical Centre and expand their premises to incorporate more
services under one roof.

▲ Question 8: On-call accommodation

*We are finding it difficult to attract locums who will work at
weekends at our practice. There seems to be a dearth of doctors
available to do this work in our area. How can we attract candidates
from further afield?*

In order to entice doctors who live at some distance from the
practice to provide locum cover at night or at weekends for the

practice, you would stand a better chance if you were able to offer on-call accommodation. If there is a room in the surgery or, better still, a separate flat which you can offer to a locum then this might make all the difference. You will then be able to advertise much more widely and might find a doctor from many miles distant who, for personal reasons, would be happy to spend some time in your practice area and undertake locum work on the condition that accommodation was provided. I know of one practice who managed to entice a retired GP from many miles away for occasional weekends on-call because following his tour of duty, he was glad to be able to see something of his married daughter who lived only a few miles from the surgery.

If you do not have a room that is suitable, do you have a community hospital close by who would be willing to rent a small on-call room to a locum? If so, you might suggest to any interested doctor that you would be prepared to pay the charge for this (it is unlikely to be very much). The added advantage of this arrangement is that the doctor making visits in an unknown area while on night duty can draw on the local knowledge of the nurses working at the hospital on night duty for directions.

More doctors in recent years are electing to do locum work for a period of time rather than tie themselves down to one practice before they are sure of their future plans. Locum work can be lucrative, although there are the inevitable gaps in employment, and it has the added advantage of infinite flexibility. However, although there are more locums, there is also a great deal more demand for their services. Therefore anything that you can do to make your practice an attractive proposition will pay dividends in the end.

▲ Question 9: Implications for premises of the shift from secondary to primary care

We read constantly in the GP press about pressure on practices caused by the introduction of more and more services to primary care from the secondary sector. Is this shift likely to continue?

Since the introduction of the new contract in 1990 GPs have been encouraged by successive governments to provide more and better services for patients within their practices. This has put a considerable strain on smaller practices who are in cramped inner-city or small town premises where the possibility of expanding is limited. Many have made the decision to move to new custom-built premises as soon as a suitable site and adequate funding became available. However, there are others who remain in unsuitable buildings where they find it difficult to offer all the services which are increasingly considered essential to a well-run practice, such as minor surgery and health promotion activities.

The shift from secondary care has included the increasing prevalence of consultant-led outreach clinics within practices, together with the transfer from hospital to surgery of services such as physiotherapy and chiropody. All these additional activities require space and it is likely that this emphasis on providing care within the community will continue. The White Paper published in December 1997 states the government's intention of increasing the co-operation between GP and community staff. By integrating primary and community health care and basing more services within GP practices and community hospitals, the devolution from large city-centre hospitals to the community seems generally set to continue.

A symposium was held at the Royal Institute of British Architects in 1996 which brought GPs and architects together to discuss the whole question of the future of practice development. One idea that was suggested involved setting up key local GP practices to deliver extended services to patients. It was hoped that these practices could then be empowered to pass the message on to other GP practices. The ultimate aim was to develop one-stop health care resource centres, based on local need and providing value-for-money health care services. The general consensus that arose out of the symposium was that GP premises should be more accommodating, accessible and adaptable. A pilot scheme is being developed in Knowle in Bristol, an area with a high level of deprivation, which is planned along the lines discussed. The development includes ideas such as a leisure centre and crèche as well as all the usual medical facilities and access to physiotherapy, chiropody and complementary therapists.

Any practice which is currently in cramped premises should be trying to find a way to increase the amount of space available, even if it means moving to larger premises rather than expanding those they already have. Ways of financing such a move are discussed in answer to a separate question (*see* Question **22**).

▲ Question 10: Outreach clinics

How do practices manage to provide specialized equipment in order to have consultant-run outpatient clinics in their surgeries?

In the main, practices do not attempt to provide all the specialized equipment which certain specialties might require in order to examine patients. However, there are some specialties, such as dermatology, gynaecology, general surgery and audiology, which do not generally require access to expensive equipment, particularly for the initial appointment and usually for many of the follow-up appointments following surgery also. The patients can benefit from services provided close to home and do not have to travel to the nearest large hospital which, in rural areas, can be many miles distant.

Where special equipment is required, the league of friends or patient participation group in the practice might be persuaded to raise funds locally in order to purchase special medical equipment for the use of patients. It is usual for such equipment to be presented to the practice on permanent loan by the group, who are likely to have charitable status and therefore be unable to donate items outright.

Fundholding practices have on occasions obtained permission from their health authority to spend savings from the previous year's budget on certain equipment such as slit lamps, hydraulic couches, endoscopes and sigmoidoscopes. Such equipment enables the GPs to provide specialized services within the practice for their own patients as well as for others.

▲ Question 11: Subletting to other practitioners

We have some rooms in our surgery which we do not use and which we are considering renting out to other practitioners. Can you tell me what would be a reasonable rent and to which kind of practitioners we could consider letting the rooms?

It is entirely up to the partners as to which particular practitioners they wish to have on the premises. They will obviously want to consider the possibility that patients will see the presence of such practitioners within the surgery as an endorsement by the GPs of their complementary medicine. It is therefore important that the partners agree among themselves just which therapies they would consider acceptable. For instance, many GPs are not yet convinced of the proven efficacy of reflexology and so might prefer not to give space to a reflexologist at this stage. However, there are currently many complementary therapists and others practising in surgeries including physiotherapists, homoeopaths, hypnotherapists, psychotherapists, counsellors, podiatrists and chiropodists as well as specialists offering acupuncture, chiro-practic and osteopathy. Any of these might make suitable tenants.

Other possibilities, depending on the sort of space you have available, would be a pharmacist, an optician or a dentist. These latter would be able and, indeed, probably willing to pay a rather higher rent than the other therapists but in return they would also certainly require more space and possibly other facilities such as a reception and message-taking service.

Whatever you decide, you should remember that if you are in receipt of cost or notional rent, this will almost certainly be reduced by the health authority if you are renting out surplus space within your practice and receiving payment from other sources. If you make a charge only for expenses incurred such as heat, light, cleaning and reception service, this should not affect your rental payments from the health authority. So be aware that you will need to take this into consideration when negotiating a satisfactory agreement.

▲ Question 12: Primary Care Groups

The latest White Paper mentions primary care groups and suggests that GPs and community nurses will be required to work together to plan patient services. How is the new system likely to develop?

The government is keen to integrate primary care with community trusts. One aim is to improve liaison between community staff and general practitioners in order to minimize any overlap in services provided and to reduce costs accordingly. Fundholding will be phased out gradually from April 1999 and primary care groups will be set up which will consist of GPs and community staff representing up to 100 000 patients.

These primary care groups will be accountable to health autho-rities and will be required to work within a 'health improvement programme'. Such programmes will be jointly agreed between health authorities, NHS trusts, the primary care groups themselves and other primary care professionals. No statement has been made as to who will arbitrate when the inevitable competing interests become apparent.

Targets for improving health services and value for money will be set and there will be an emphasis on audit with a view to improving provision of care within the community. Members of the primary care group will be expected to spearhead any improvements identified as being required within the locality. A senior professional within the group – not necessarily a GP – will take the lead on standards generally and on planning professional development within the group.

It is felt that these groups who work closely with patients in the community are likely to be best qualified to determine just which services are required. The hope is that the GPs and nurses in such groups will continue to demand responsiveness from hospital trusts to local needs and to extend the range of services available within their own individual surgeries. The White Paper states that 'Primary care groups will grow out of the range of commissioning models that have developed in recent years but will give a sharper focus to their work'. There will be less money (£3 per patient) and less flexibility for individual practices compared to their experiences under the fundholding scheme. The challenge will be to get the practices who previously relished the opportunity for innovative provision of services that fundholding status gave to use the negotiating and commissioning skills they gained to help in the formation of successful primary care groups.

▲ Question 13: Community staff

I understand that the recent White Paper has stressed the need for GPs and community nurses to be the prime movers in forming primary care groups. How is this development likely to affect our practice and in particular, the possible need to accommodate community staff?

One of the aims of the primary care groups, as set out in the 1997 White Paper, is to shift more of the responsibility for providing and commissioning patient services on to GPs in co-operation with the community nurses (*see* Question **12**). This working relationship between GPs and nurses may not be without problems as doctors and community staff are both likely to be reluctant to surrender their hard-fought battle for autonomy to such a partnership. Currently some community nurses are attached to more than one practice which means that their contact with individual GPs can be spasmodic and unreliable. Many have their base outside the surgery itself and this can cause problems of communication between doctors and nurses looking after their patients in the community. It would seem probable that it will become increasingly convenient for community staff to be based within general practice premises wherever possible.

The way forward will be for community nurses attached to a specific practice to have an office within the surgery, if they do not do so already. Messages taken for them can then be relayed more effectively by practice staff and liaison with GPs should be relatively simple during the working day when individual patients need to be discussed.

By its very nature, a lot of the district nurses' work is done in the community but there are times each day when they need to write up notes or reports and use the telephone. It is helpful if their office can be within the practice in these circumstances. The community trust that employs them should provide any equipment such as telephone, computers and office furniture and should be willing to pay a nominal charge for the use of the room. However, you should not overlook the fact that if you accept a commercial rent for the space, you will have to inform the health authority and it is likely that any cost rent or notional rent that you currently receive for that part of the building will be adjusted accordingly. It is sometimes simpler to settle for a service charge to cover the cost of heat, light, cleaning and staff time in message taking as this will not affect rental reimbursements from the health authority.

Close co-operation is certainly easier if staff can meet on a daily basis, however informally, to discuss particular problems or cases. GPs will have to delegate more and more of the routine treatment of their patients in the community to nurses as patient demand for health care increases generally. The pressure on general practices to incorporate more and more services is unlikely to decrease in the foreseeable future and if you can make provision for accommodating community staff in your practice now, this would seem to be a wise move.

▲ Question 14: Nurse treatment rooms

We are planning to revamp our nurse treatment room. What particular points should we be considering?

An increasing number of different tasks are now being undertaken in nurse treatment rooms following the decision of many GPs to delegate more work to their nurses. Often a small team of part-time practice nurses works within the practice providing all the necessary services of immunizations, inoculations, cervical smears, leg ulcer treatments and health promotion clinics. Patients value privacy and it is important that wherever possible, patients should not be overheard when consulting a nurse. This means that curtained cubicles, although providing a degree of privacy, are not ideal and a closed door is the preferred option. Thus if two nurses are working simultaneously – as often happens – then two rooms will be necessary. Both do not need to have the full range of equipment, however. A hydraulic couch is essential in one room for smears and other treatments necessitating the patient lying prone. However, a chair is probably sufficient in the room where the nurses mostly undertake childhood or flu inoculations, travel immunizations and ear syringeing.

Any treatment room should have a non-slip floor that is easy to clean, preferably of some vinyl that has no seams. If the floor surface can be continued for several inches up the wall this prevents germs settling in any cracks at the edges of the room. Wipe-clean surfaces are obviously essential throughout and lockable cupboard doors for supplies should be standard. Chairs should not be on castors. All equipment should be well maintained, particularly such items as the autoclave which has to be serviced regularly in order to comply with health and safety regulations. Sharps bins should be available at each workstation and clinical waste should be stored in separate containers from the ordinary waste paper.

It is probably helpful to visit one or two neighbouring practices to see if they have come up against any snags in the planning of their treatment rooms. Why reinvent the wheel? By talking to the nurses working in other surgeries, you may avoid some of the more common problems encountered in treatment room design.

▲ Question 15: Soundproof consulting rooms

We have had one or two complaints from patients who believe that details of their consultation were overheard by others waiting outside the consulting room. How can we improve matters and ensure privacy for our patients?

Safeguarding confidentiality is becoming more of a problem as services are devolved to general practice and there is pressure to increase the space available and also to maximize the usage of existing rooms. This pressure for space has often meant that nurses are having to use treatment rooms only divided by a curtain or screen from others. These flimsy partitions create an illusion of privacy but in fact all conversations are audible to those on the other side.

Older buildings often have solid doors but may have thin partition walls dividing up the original large rooms. Modern buildings are more likely to have sound insulation built in but it is not always as effective as was originally hoped. An obvious way of ensuring that conversations within a consulting room are less likely to be overheard by patients sitting outside is to distance the waiting patients some way from the doctor's room if at all possible. A second door with a small hallway between consulting room and waiting area is one way of achieving this. Rearranging the chairs to ensure that none is close to the door would be helpful. Another solution might be to have music or 'white noise' playing which masks all but the loudest conversations.

Another area of concern should be open windows in treatment rooms or consulting rooms. Care must be taken to lessen the possibility that people walking past will overhear conversations. One idea I have heard suggested is that a small electric fan be placed in the window to create sufficient noise to provide privacy. I rather suspect that if the level of noise were high enough to drown out the sound of voices, then it would almost certainly also interfere with the conversation within the room. Again, distancing the passers-by from the immediate vicinity of the open windows would seem to be a better solution, if possible.

▲ Question 16: Child health clinic

Since the introduction of targets for childhood immunizations and the need for the GPs to undertake child health surveillance, we have set aside one afternoon a week for our practice nurse to run a child health clinic. What can we do to increase the take-up of such services?

The new contract in 1990 certainly helped to raise awareness of the need for special clinics for certain target groups. In particular, the increasing percentage of babies now having their full course of immunizations by the age of two has been dramatic and welcomed by parents and GPs alike. However, scares such as the recent one about a possible link between MMR vaccine and subsequent autism can mean that parents are unwilling to take up the offer of immunization for their babies. It can sometimes be a good idea to elicit the help of health visitors in an approach to such parents. Health visitors are in touch with the parents of all children under five within the practice and so they would seem well placed to help persuade those reluctant to bring their children for immunization.

Health visitors in some practices have set up regular weekly clinics where mothers with their babies can discuss any problems. This system has many advantages over the time-consuming individual home visiting previously undertaken by community staff. It allows parents to meet others with children the same age and to share solutions to common problems. It also means that the GP or practice nurse can approach the parent opportunistically and offer overdue immunizations for the babies. Health visitors are able to provide health education to the group of mothers and babies on a regular basis and this can include topical information. For instance, if there has been a recent case of meningitis in the area, the health visitors have an ideal forum for advising parents on the tell-tale signs to look out for and when they should call their GP.

By running such clinics which include the health visitors, the practice will possibly attract more mothers and babies to the practice on a regular basis.

▲ Question 17: Car parking

Patients are finding it difficult to park in the vicinity of the practice. The practice car park has only a limited number of spaces and doctors and staff fill many of these. Have you any suggestions as to how we can overcome this problem?

Many town centre or city practices have this problem. One of the obvious ways of releasing spaces is to ask staff not to bring their cars to work or, if they must, to park them elsewhere. Staff will almost certainly protest, since free parking is considered to be a useful perk in any job. However, if you are really pressed for space this is an obvious first step. You can sweeten the pill by offering to make a contribution towards the cost of public transport or bicycle repairs for any member of staff who uses one of these alternative means of transport. You could also offer to cover a proportion of the parking charges that staff would have to pay if they choose to continue driving to work but now have to park elsewhere in a commercial car park.

If there are still insufficient spaces for patients to use when visiting the surgery, you could approach your local council and see if they would allow the surgery to lease spaces in a nearby council car park on an annual basis specifically for the use of patients. It is important that those who use the surgery car park are genuinely visiting the practice and that the system is not abused. If you choose this option, you might like to prepare windscreen stickers which can be placed prominently on any car found to be parking inappropriately. Some practices have resorted to buying a wheel-clamp to place on offending vehicles. Others have resorted to the simple expedient of getting one of the doctors to double-park the offending car so that the owner has to come to reception to beg for release! If the doctor is with a patient in surgery, the motorist might have to wait some time to escape which should help to make the point that the parking spaces are private.

An afterthought. Are patients being kept waiting for an inordinate amount of time to see their GP or nurse in the practice? Would a revamp of the appointment system be a worthwhile exercise in order to speed up the turnover of patients, reducing waiting times and the inevitable overlap and thus easing at least some of the parking problems?

▲ Question 18: Staff rest areas

We do not have set coffee breaks in our practice. At the moment staff just make a cup of coffee when they can spare the time and drink it at their desk. I feel this is not very satisfactory but we are really pushed for space. Any suggestions?

Break times are essential in any job and particularly in a setting as stressful as a busy surgery. Receptionists need a chance to escape from the desk and the demands of patients and doctors alike. They need to have the opportunity to renew their energies. It is also important that they have a chance to chat to each other informally when not actually working. This socializing helps individuals to feel part of the team. Mugs of coffee at the reception desk do not give a good impression to callers and there is always the danger of liquid being spilt over vital computer equipment or papers.

If you have no separate room that can be set aside for use as a staffroom, is there any space that could be converted for this use? Perhaps a room that is not in constant occupation could be used for this purpose just at break times or during the lunch hour? Staff and GPs in some smaller practices use the same common room, but usually at different times. This can work although it is important to ensure that doctors and staff alike have time on their own so that they can really relax.

Obviously staff will have to stagger their break times to ensure that the telephones and reception area are constantly attended. It is helpful if any secretarial, nursing or managerial staff have varying break times too, thus mixing with different members of staff on each day. It is surprising how often potential problems are raised during these informal discussions which can be solved before they become a major concern.

▲ Question 19: Partner in charge

Our senior partner prefers to take responsibility for the supervision of all areas of management of the practice. The problem is that we are currently considering expanding the premises and he has little time in which to discuss important issues with me. What should I do?

It is not unusual for the senior partner to wish to retain control over his practice. The likelihood is that he has worked many years in the same practice and feels somewhat proprietorial about its management. However, with the increasing pressures on GPs' time it is unlikely that he will be able to supervise all aspects of management including staff, finances, clinical protocols, premises and information technology.

Many partnerships have allocated these various tasks between all the partners, perhaps rotating the roles every few years. It makes sense that the most computer-literate GP supervises all the information technology in the practice and the doctor most knowledgeable about the finances oversees all aspects of the accounting. The manager is also likely to need support when making decisions on the maintenance of the building and redecoration of the premises. It is helpful to have one partner with whom she can liaise when problems do occur.

It would be wise to discuss the idea of individual partner responsibility with the doctors at the next partners' meeting and see if you can obtain their agreement to working in this way. You could stress that no major decision would be made without prior referral to a meeting of all the partners so the senior partner could be assured that he would not lose control of the practice. However, he would be able to devote more time to medicine and less to management, which is most GPs' dream, and his partners might feel they have a greater stake in the practice by taking on individual responsibility for supervision of a particular area of management. It would also enable them to build up some expertise in the chosen field, whether it be management of staff, buildings, technology or finance.

▲ Question 20: Cost rent/notional rent

Please can you explain the difference between cost rent and notional rent? Do we have a choice as to which to apply for?

These two schemes are described in detail in section 51 of the Statement of Fees and Allowances (SFA). Qualifying criteria are complex but basically the two schemes are as follows.

Cost rent is paid by the health authority for new surgeries, ones that are acquired which require substantial modification or for existing practice premises which need major alterations. The health authority has to determine priorities when allocating cost rent, as it is cash limited and so before entering into any financial commitment, it is essential that the practice obtains a written offer from the health authority confirming that the proposed project will be acceptable for reimbursement on a cost rent basis, together with a target date for commencement of payments. The cost schedules in the SFA specify the upper limits on what the authority will pay for new separate purpose-built premises or their equivalent. The number of rooms need not equal the number of partners as consideration will be given to provision of accommodation for a GP registrar and community staff. The White Paper published in December 1996, entitled *Primary Care: Delivering the Future*, proposed the introduction of new, more generous cost rent schedules that take into account the fact that more and more services are being shifted to primary care and therefore the requirement for accommodation is likely to be greater.

The cost rent scheme, which is cash limited, is designed to help practices pay the interest on loans taken out to fund the building project. New, more generous cost rent schedules were introduced in 1997 which enable GPs to build and develop much larger buildings than previously. Areas such as the cost of security measures can be included for the first time. The schedules will be reviewed annually in April. The cost rent allowance does not represent the actual interest paid on the loan and any shortfall should be kept to a minimum as the GPs will have to make this up themselves out of profits.

A key feature of the cost rent scheme is the recognition of the difference in the actual cost of the building project and its true market value, which is invariably substantially lower at the outset. It is calculated using the variable reimbursement rate notified by the DoH on approved costs actually incurred in the project. If the GPs are financing the scheme mainly through a loan on a fixed rate basis or are using their own money to finance the loan, the prescribed percentage will be the fixed reimbursement rate.

Notional rent, on the other hand, is paid to GPs who own their own surgeries which are neither new nor recently developed under the cost rent scheme. Notional rent is based on the current market rent as assessed by a district valuer taking into account its function as a medical centre. Notional rent is not cash limited but it is advisable to enter into discussions with the health authority at an early stage if the partners are considering a switch from cost to notional rent.

Rent is usually paid quarterly by the health authority and is reviewed every three years. It is possible to contest a district valuer's assessment of the current market value of your property if you feel that he or she has undervalued the building. The rules regarding valuation of surgeries have changed recently and they are now valued as medical centres, rather than just as commercial buildings. If you decide to contest the valuation, you would be wise to consult a valuer who has knowledge of local conditions who will assess the value himself and help you in your negotiations regarding the original valuation.

When deciding on whether the time is right to switch from cost rent to notional rent, you should do your sums carefully. Once you have switched to notional rent, the decision is irrevocable. A careful assessment of the likely direction of interest rates is therefore crucial before such a decision is made.

▲ Question 21: Health centre leasing

We are being encouraged to sign a lease on our health centre premises. What facts should we be aware of before signing such a lease?

There are two types of lease currently available for GPs leasing health centres. The GMSC and the NHS have both produced forms of lease to cater for the ongoing occupation by GPs of health authority-owned premises. Health authorities are usually keen to divest themselves of the responsibility for the maintenance costs of such premises and are increasingly encouraging GPs to buy or lease long term the health centres in which they practise. The DoH has issued a recommended form of lease and the GMSC has produced another.

Before making any decision on which form of lease to sign, the partners should first consider whether they wish to remain in the premises at all. Signing a lease would tie them to remaining there for 20 years. If they are keen to remain and are willing to plan for the long term, they should be considering purchasing the freehold of the property in order to give themselves more scope in the future.

There are two kinds of leasing: one under which the tenant is prepared to accept full repairing and insurance (FRI) liability and the other in which they are only responsible for internal repairing liability. If you are considering the former, you should have a full structural survey done and a 'schedule of condition' should be agreed. This would then ensure that the partners could not be required at some future date to put the premises into a better state of repair than they were in when first acquired.

Lawyers seem in some doubt about what the NHS and GMSC leases require but it is assumed that the NHS lease imposes FRI liability, whereas the GMSC lease only requires internal repairing. Both leases provide for a service charge for repair of common parts. However, the NHS lease provides for a fixed percentage according to the user of the premises, while a percentage of occupancy is what the GMSC lease stipulates. As the occupancy levels could vary during the term of the lease, this might provide greater flexibility.

If the GPs so wish, the NHS lease permits alterations to be made with the landlord's consent. However, the GMSC lease prohibits any modifications although the landlord may be prevented from refusing if such alterations are 'consistent with the permitted use'.

It is important to be certain for what exact period the partners are committing themselves when signing the lease. Either party can break the NHS lease on the tenth anniversary of the form although if an improvement grant has been received, this option might be limited. The GMSC lease is rather more flexible, permitting either party to withdraw at any time after the first year, although the landlord is obliged to give 24 months' notice if the tenant is a sole practitioner. Rent reviews will occur every three years under the NHS lease and every five years under the GMSC scheme.

There are many factors to take into account when considering leasing a health centre and it is essential that the partners should consult a solicitor for clarification of any lease before signing.

▲ Question 22: Obtaining funds to build premises

We are planning to extend our premises in the near future and seek guidance on how we should go about obtaining the required finance.

Answers to other questions in this book give details of various options regarding expanding practice premises. These include siting satellite surgeries within a superstore development or high street pharmacy (*see* Questions **5** and **6**). However, if you are looking for funding of an extension to your present premises the partners are going to have to approach the health authority with a view to discussing cost rent. This is designed to help practices to pay the interest on loans taken out to cover the cost of their building projects. It is not a direct reimbursement of the actual interest paid on the loan. However, the scheme does recognize that there is a difference in the cost of building and its true market value, the market value invariably being substantially lower at the outset (*see* Question **20**).

Income under the cost rent scheme is often less than the actual cost of servicing the debt, the amount paid being based on a figure that the DoH considers to be a reasonable average level of return on capital. This inevitably means that the practice will suffer from negative equity from the start and it is therefore vital that your lender is informed of the intricacies of the cost rent scheme when you are negotiating a loan.

Most practices will borrow money to fund building schemes from a bank, building society or insurance company. The General Practice Finance Corporation (GPFC), which is now part of Norwich Union, specializes in lending to GPs but so do certain banks, notably the TSB and the Royal Bank of Scotland. The bank where the practice has their account would probably be willing to consider financing the project, given the guarantee of cost rent reimbursement. However, there may not necessarily be a cost rent specialist in your local branch and so it is important that when approaching a bank for a loan, a good case is made with clear explanation of the cost rent scheme.

The partners will have to decide whether they wish to take out a fixed or variable rate loan. This will depend both on their individual circumstances and the economic climate that prevails at the time. The partners should seek expert advice before committing themselves to any specific loan arrangements.

GPs negotiating a large loan on their practice premises should ensure that they have a good partnership agreement, in which arrangements for the cost rent project are drawn up carefully to protect each of the partners as far as possible against potential problems with negative equity. A partner retiring within a few years or wishing to reduce their commitment and work part time would require careful adjustments to be made to the way the capital is distributed and responsibility for repaying it allocated. Provision for this should also be made in the partnership agreement.

The question of negative equity, touched on briefly above, is a major factor in new partners' decision to buy into the practice or not. Many are refusing to buy in at the inflated mortgaged value when the current market value is considerably less. The other partners should make allowances for this natural reluctance and perhaps permit the new partner to wait several years before buying into a share of the premises. In the meantime some financial arrangement would have to be made whereby the cost rent payments are divided in the property ownership share ratios rather than between all the partners equally.

▲ Question 23: Bank loans

We are going to approach our bank for a loan to fund the purchase of an expensive piece of equipment that the partners require. How can we get the best deal?

The first thing to realize when approaching the bank for a loan is that the practice is likely to be a favoured customer. It is very rare for a general practice to go bankrupt and of course a large percentage of a GP's income is guaranteed by the health authority so they are unlikely to renege on any deal. The bank manager will therefore be reluctant to lose the practice custom and is likely to offer good rates for any loan for which the practice can offer adequate security. It should therefore be possible to negotiate a rate lower than the normal commercial rate set for other, more risky businesses.

If you have no luck with your own bank in negotiating a rate only one or two points above base rate (rather than the more common three or four points offered to other businesses), it might be worth approaching other banks in the area to see if they would be prepared to offer a better rate were the practice to move its business to them. If nothing else, this might provide you with competitive quotes which would give you the required ammunition to approach your own bank once again. They will not want to lose the practice account, for the reasons given above. Also, most practices have large amounts of money paid into their accounts on a regular basis and many are not always scrupulous in transferring surplus funds immediately to interest-bearing accounts. This is naturally to the bank's advantage and adds to the attraction of GP practices as customers.

▲ Question 24: Improvement grants

How do we go about seeking an improvement grant for extending our present practice premises?

First you will need to seek prior approval from your health authority for any improvements to the surgery that you wish to make. The improvement grant budget is necessarily limited and there is fierce competition for any funds that are available. Consequently you may not be offered a grant at all, however good your case, if the health authority has already allocated the whole of the budget available for the coming year.

Grants can represent anything from one-third to two-thirds of the cost (including VAT) of the project, including professional fees associated with both the design and the supervision of the work. Local authority fees for inspecting the building and passing the plans can be included in the total project costs.

Extending or adapting the premises in order to provide a minor surgery room, improve wheelchair access, adapt a lavatory for the use of disabled people or add extra rooms to accommodate attached staff (provided no rent is charged) are all projects likely to be considered eligible for an improvement grant, if there are funds available.

There are strict criteria for eligibility and you should read section 56 of the Statement of Fees and Allowances (SFA) for the details. You should be aware that if you subsequently apply for cost rent on the project, according to the Red Book 'The amount of any improvement grant paid will be deducted from the aggregate cost to which the prescribed percentage is applied'.

▲ Question 25: Private financing

What is the PFI which is mentioned in connection with building GP premises?

PFI stands for the Private Finance Initiative which was intended to enable GPs to obtain funding from developers for their practice premises. Currently, it means that the developer takes all the risk but also retains the reward of owning the surgery themselves. The GPs merely pay rent and run their business offering health care in a building that someone else owns. They would not therefore have the opportunity to benefit from any capital appreciation, unlike GPs who own their own practice premises. Until recently, owner-occupying GPs have found that this has been of considerable benefit on retirement. However, with recent falls in the value of premises the question of negative equity has rather blighted the situation, particularly in respect of new partners who are naturally reluctant to buy into a building for an amount higher than the current market value.

Valerie Martin, National Director of Medical Services at

Pannell Kerr Forster, speaking at the symposium on Future Premises for Primary Health Care held in 1996, claimed that if PFI were a real private finance initiative, the developer would not only own the surgery but would also run it as well. She stated that PFI is useful if doctors do not wish to own their premises – for instance, if they were planning a large-scale health care centre. A PFI-funded scheme would permit the GPs to 'concentrate on providing medical services while somebody else owned and ran the enterprise'.

However, historically GPs have benefited from the capital appreciation of the premises they own and it is probable that they will continue to wish to own their own premises whenever feasible. It is unlikely that they will be willing to lose the opportunity for benefiting from capital appreciation when they retire, other than in exceptional circumstances.

▲ Question 26: Endowment mortgages

I understand from a lender that endowment mortgages are no longer the ideal way of borrowing money on private property. Does this apply to loans covering GP surgeries also?

No, it does not. Endowment policies are still the best bet for borrowing on practice premises because of the tax relief at the higher rate that most GPs receive on any interest paid to the lender. This tax relief would not be payable on capital repayments, of course. Although the partners will still have to pay tax on the cost rent payments received from the health authority, at least they start from the advantage of having some tax relief to offset against the tax due.

▲ Question 27: Valuations

Our premises were valued recently and the valuation is much lower than we had anticipated. Can we dispute this valuation placed on our property by the health authority for calculation of notional rent?

The district valuer values a GP's premises for the health authority and decides on the rental payments he considers appropriate for reimbursement. However, if you feel the premises have been undervalued, you can employ your own valuer to give a second opinion. You should make sure that the valuer you choose has a good working knowledge of local conditions and the going rental rates in the area. Recent changes in the rules have meant that the building is valued as a medical centre, rather than as a commercial property. His valuation, if it is more than that of the district valuer, as is likely, can be used in any negotiations you have with the health authority for the calculation of notional rent payments.

In one particular practice, the two valuations were tens of thousands of pounds apart and the increase in notional rent which was negotiated amounted to almost 50% more than the original figure offered. It is therefore well worth seeking a second opinion if you are in any doubt as to the accuracy of the district valuer's figures.

▲ Question 28: Building and contents insurance

How often should we look at our insurance cover and how do we know whether we are paying a reasonable premium?

You should review the level of insurance cover on the practice premises and contents annually. Points you will need to go through are similar to those you would consider when renewing your own home insurance. You should of course bear in mind that the value of the premises is that of the cost of rebuilding and not the likely sale value. Have any major changes been made to the premises during the past year which might add to its likely value?

Contents cover should be kept up-to-date also. It is helpful to make an inventory room by room of all furniture and equipment and to amend this when items are replaced or renewed. Many managers are surprised at just how much expensive equipment they have in their practices. The staff kitchen alone might house a refrigerator, a microwave, a washing machine, a tumble drier, electric kettles, a coffee maker and water filter. The nurses' treatment room will probably have an autoclave, hydraulic couch, ophthalmoscopes, sphygmomanometers, stethoscopes and various supplies and vaccines. In the case of total loss, whether by fire or flood, the cost of replacing all these items can be considerable.

Some practices are finding it necessary to take out cover against terrorist attack, others against an in-depth tax investigation. The kind of cover you require will depend where your practice is located and what you believe the risks to be. An investigation by the Inland Revenue can be very costly in time alone and some practices have felt it advisable to offset the likely costs by taking out insurance just in case their practice is highlighted for investigation.

Once you have worked out the probable cost of replacement should a fire destroy everything, you should then ring around various companies for a quotation. If you can show that you have calculated the likely replacement costs of all the equipment and rebuilding costs of the premises, companies will be able to give you an accurate quote. These can then be compared and you can use specific quotations to negotiate with your preferred insurer. Be aware that the cheapest insurance cover is not always the best.

▲ Question 29: Security

Our practice is located near the centre of a large city and the premises have been broken into several times in the past few years. Can you suggests ways in which we can improve the security of the premises?

The security of practice premises is becoming an increasing problem for GPs. A recent article in *GP* stated that 40% of practices had been targets of crime over the previous three months. The statistics included threatening and abusive behaviour from violent patients but the majority of incidents involved theft of equipment or damage to property. Anything that delays entry or departure from the building increases the chance of a burglar being caught. The average thief leaves the premises within four minutes, often having smashed his way in and out, grabbing items of high value which are easily portable.

Solid doors, window locks, bars and wrought iron grilles are worth considering as they act as a deterrent although they are unlikely to prevent the really determined thief. They might perhaps delay him long enough for any electronic device to alert the police or neighbours. However, architects undertaking a security survey of new premises are now recommending double or even triple glazing as being more effective than bars or grilles. Installation of reflective glass on all downstairs windows is a good idea as it prevents potential thieves from prying. Flat roofs provide an easy point of entry and a pitched roof is obviously preferable if at all possible.

In some areas closed circuit cameras are a sensible precaution and pictures from this can be relayed to a monitor in reception. The camera itself can act as a visual deterrent to a would-be thief and of course dummy cameras, if they are sufficiently convincing, can be effective although you are advised to have at least one real camera, providing visible monitoring within the building.

You may decide to have an intruder alarm linked to the local police station or one that just makes an audible alarm sound when a detection circuit has been breached. It is possible to cover specific doorways, such as those leading to drug stores or computer rooms, with these devices. Providing combination locks on internal doors and ensuring that these are locked at night or when the rooms are empty can act as another tactic for delaying would-be thieves.

Computers rather than drugs are often the target for thieves today and ways of minimizing theft of computers or microchips are discussed in answer to the question on computer security (*see* Question **70**) in the section on information technology.

If you are in any doubt about how you can improve the security of your practice, you should ask the police for advice. The local crime prevention officer will make suggestions and will almost certainly be able to give you a list of approved local security firms whom you can approach for further help. Your insurer might be willing to sponsor a security survey when an expert can give you sound advice on ways in which you can make your particular premises more secure and protect practice property.

▲ Question 30: Safeguards against violent patients

Are there any inexpensive ways in which we can adapt our premises in order to reduce the possibility of doctors or staff being assaulted by the occasional violent patient?

The incidence of violent patients in general practice is sadly increasing. Practices are having to take this into account when designing the layout of their premises and are also having to adjust staff rotas so that there is sufficient cover to ensure the personal safety of staff and doctors.

In order to keep an illusion of openness at reception, which most practices are anxious to do, adapting the reception desk itself may help to avoid the use of screens or grilles. If you find that

irate patients can lean over the reception desk to attack receptionists, the easiest solution might be to widen and heighten the desk
so that the patient is unable to reach the person standing behind.
If you do this in a two-tier construction there should also be room
underneath the front section for filing trays or computer screens.
This should provide sufficient protection without being so high as
to prevent shorter patients being able to see over. A suggested
height is 125 cm which is about chest height on the average
person.

Panic buttons in consulting rooms and at reception are useful
and can help doctors and staff feel more secure, particularly when
working with a skeleton staff in the evenings or at a weekend.

There are training courses in diffusing potentially violent situa-
tions available with an emphasis on negotiation. However, staff
might feel safer if they also underwent some training in basic self-
defence.

If all else fails and you have a particularly difficult patient, one
practice in Buckinghamshire found a solution to the problem.
The man had been struck off the list of all the local practices and
was having to be allocated to GPs in turn in order to receive
treatment. After several instances of staff being threatened and
one incident where he threw a brick through the practice
manager's window, the GP finally stated that he would only see
the patient if he was in custody in a police cell in the town. The
health authority, the LMC and the local police force agreed to
this unusual solution. It meant that the patient no longer turned
up at the surgery (or any other in the area) unannounced and out
to cause trouble but could still be sure of receiving medical
treatment when really necessary.

▲ Question 31: Fire precautions

*We recently invited the fire prevention officer to look round our
premises and advise on ways in which we could improve them as*

regards fire safety. We plan to make the changes he advised. What else should we be doing?

Now that you presumably have the requisite number of fire doors in place and fire exits clearly marked, you must ensure that the staff are adequately trained in how to evacuate the building safely.

You should have regular fire drills, preferably when there are patients within the building, during which staff will follow a protocol using designated exits, checking specific areas and assembling at a safe point outside the building. You will need to take a printed copy of the appointments if one is to hand so that names of patients can be checked off against this. All rooms including examination rooms and lavatories should be checked by a member of staff and any patients escorted safely out of the building. If a fire drill is held regularly (once a month seems ideal) then in the event of a real fire, everything should run smoothly.

In addition to staff training in fire drills, there is a statutory requirement for you to test fire alarm bells regularly. You should ensure this is done and a note should be kept in a special log of the date and time of each test. The alarm system should be regularly maintained by a recognized engineer.

The fire prevention officer will recommend the siting of fire extinguishers and will explain to you the different types you will need to have. For instance, fires in electrical equipment require a dry powder extinguisher, rather than a water one which would only exacerbate the situation. It is important that these are placed appropriately and not used to prop open fire doors. These extinguishers should be serviced annually and a note kept of dates of service. As extinguishers get old they will need to be replaced and the service engineer will tell you when this is likely to be. His company may be able to supply a new one, but you should ring around other local companies for competitive prices before committing yourself to buy.

▲ Question 32: Disposal of sharps

We have an acupuncturist who works one afternoon a week in our surgery. The cleaner was upset to find used needles lying under the couch on several occasions following his sessions. What should we do?

It is important that a sharps bin is made available in the consulting room for the use of the acupuncturist. You should inform him/her that stray needles have been found on the floor and stress the importance of careful disposal. He/she should be asked to count needles out as they are placed in patients and to account for each one at the end of the treatment session.

Sharps containers should be collected and exchanged regularly by a specialist company approved by the health authority. The cleaner should be made aware of the need to wear gloves at all times when cleaning rooms used by clinicians. The risk of touching used needles or other clinical waste without adequate protection should be clearly pointed out.

▲ Question 33: Health and safety issues

How do health and safety issues affect those working in general practice? What should I be doing to safeguard staff and patients?

There are no shortcuts. For a start, you will have to obtain a copy of the Control of Substances Hazardous to Health Regulations (COSHH) from the Health and Safety Executive and read up on how the practice should be dealing with hazardous substances. These are of relevance not only to the nursing staff but also to the cleaner. Simple things, like ensuring that no toxic substances such as cleaning materials and bleach are within reach of small children, are a start. A special protocol for dealing with spillage of hazardous waste such as blood or urine samples is essential and this should be drawn up in co-operation with the nursing staff as it will be mainly for their protection. The fear of HIV or hepatitis infection is very real for clinicians everywhere these days.

It is important to maintain the temperature of any building. A practice should be at least 16°C because of the need for patients to undress for examination. This is also a comfortable temperature for sedentary staff such as secretaries and computer operators. Adequate ventilation is also important and if there are no windows that can be opened in a room, then mechanical ventilation systems should be provided and regularly maintained.

Lighting levels should be sufficient to enable people to work and move about safely. Electrical equipment should be regularly maintained to a recognized standard. Any accidents involving staff or patients should be entered in an accident book which should be kept in an easily accessible place near the reception area.

Leaflets on *Workplace Health and Safety Welfare, Preventing Slips, Trips and Falls at Work, Manual Handling* and *Violence at Work* are all available from the Health and Safety Executive. You should obtain copies of these leaflets and once you have read them, compile your own safety policy statement for staff. Each employee should sign to say that they have been given a copy of this statement and any new members of staff should have one included with their contract of employment. The policy statement should state the practice's general aims with regard to employees' health and safety. You might also wish to stress the importance of co-operation from staff in the implementation of the practice policy.

▲ Question 34: Maintenance of building

It is proving very expensive to pay for all the repairs which seem to be necessary for this old and rambling town centre building in which our practice is situated. Is there any way we can get help towards the cost?

The maintenance of premises is often a nightmare for GP

practices, particularly since few of the surgeries are custom built. If your premises happen to be a listed building, you can apply to the local council for a grant towards the cost of essential repairs. The disadvantage of listed building status is that you have to adhere strictly to the rules and regulations, for instance repairing a roof with appropriate roof tiles that match the originals and replacing windows with ones in keeping with the architectural style. You may not be successful in your bid for such a grant; much will depend on the current state of finances at the local council and at what time in their financial year you apply, but it is certainly worth asking.

One of the advantages of working in a general practice is that the GPs usually have a good standing in the community and local workmen are happy to help out with any maintenance work. Some practices find it helpful to pay a small retainer to a local handyman, perhaps the relative of one of the staff or patients, who is then available to do any small repairs as and when required for a reasonable charge. However, even if you put work out to tender you are likely to receive favourable quotes since there is a certain amount of kudos for any local building firm in gaining a commission to work at the local surgery.

▲ Question 35: Caretaker/maintenance person

Our practice is housed in a large, rather shabby building which seems to be in constant need of minor repairs, not least because we have suffered from a series of minor break-ins recently. One of the doctors has always been nominally in charge of the premises and likes to do the necessary repairs whenever possible. The problem is that because of pressure of work he is no longer available as often as required to keep things under control. What can I suggest as a solution to our ongoing maintenance problem without offending him?

As practices increase in size to incorporate all the additional services which are now being offered in the primary care sector, GPs are required to maintain ever-expanding buildings. If the premises are large, it might be a good idea to employ a caretaker who could not only maintain the building but also help to ensure its security. Depending on the size of the practice and level of crime in the area, you could employ someone full or part time. Their duties might include simple do-it-yourself projects such as maintenance of the plumbing and heating system, redecoration and repairs both inside and out and ensuring that fire and security alarms are in working order.

It would help to make the building as user friendly as possible. For instance, providing a secure place for patients to leave prams and buggies means that they are less likely to bring them into waiting areas which can cause damage to or, at the very least, marks on walls. Heavy-duty non-slip mats which absorb dirt are a must in doorways to reduce the amount of mud walked into the building. Attention to such details in the planning of the practice should reduce the need for expensive maintenance or replacement.

If staff face frequent attack from violent patients, the caretaker could perhaps also serve as a security guard in the evenings or on Saturday mornings when fewer staff are on duty covering emergency surgeries. If there has been a spate of recent break-ins and if space permits, it would be prudent to consider employing someone to live on the premises to ensure against future attacks. One practice I know rented out a small flat on the top floor of the building at a nominal rent to a retired member of staff who kept an eye on things at night and at weekends.

It would be sensible to explain to the partners your reasons for believing that the practice needs such a person to help look after the premises. The doctor currently trying to cope with odd repairs should certainly realize that the security angle is not one he could hope to cover himself.

In order to justify the costs of employing a caretaker, even part time, you will need to prepare a record of all payments relating to redecoration and repairs paid to outside contractors over recent years and present this to the partners. You should be able to estimate how much it would cost to employ someone in-house to do the same maintenance work. Armed with the facts and figures, you could then prepare a simple feasibility study to show how, even allowing for the wages of a caretaker, savings could be made.

▲ Question 36: Decor/first impressions

Our premises are somewhat shabby. Does this really matter when the service we offer to patients is excellent?

General practice is becoming increasingly competitive as GPs attempt to expand their lists to take advantage of economies of scale. This expansion is being encouraged by the government as they devolve more and more services to GPs and away from the more expensive secondary care sector.

A recent patient survey undertaken by a practice to discover why the patient had chosen to register at this practice, found that although 30% had made their choice because of a family connection and 36% had taken account of a personal recommendation, 33% chose to register because of the location and external appearance of the surgery. There may not be much you can do to improve the location of your practice, but the external and internal appearances are important factors in attracting and retaining patients. Not only are first impressions important for visitors but working conditions can actively affect staff for good or ill also. Ask yourself some of the following questions to see if your practice makes a good first impression.

- Is the surgery clearly signed from the main street?
- Is the reception desk clearly signed?
- Is the waiting room tidy and clean?
- Is there an adequate system of patient-calling by GPs to their consulting rooms?

- Do staff appear smart and tidy?
- Do all the staff wear name badges and/or a uniform?
- Are the magazines in the waiting room tidy and up to date?
- Are any toys provided for children regularly tidied into containers?
- Is the building accessible to patients in wheelchairs or with pushchairs?
- Is there an adequate pram park?

The building should be welcoming and comfortable but also functional. It is obviously important that the nurses' treatment rooms and the doctors' consulting rooms are scrupulously clean and that matters of hygiene are taken seriously.

Good lighting can make a considerable difference to the appearance of the premises. In waiting areas the degree of lighting required will not be as great as that needed in the working areas. Pictures on the walls can be a helpful addition and if the practice does not want to go to the expense of buying paintings, a local artists' group may be happy to hang their works of art around the practice and even to make them available for sale to visitors. This arrangement can present problems if the work is not up to an agreed standard. In one practice I visited a local artist had produced a particularly ugly painting of an unprepossessing baby. The staff refused to work facing the picture and it had to be relegated to a dark corridor where it would offend few passers-by.

Some practices have music playing throughout the building which can be an advantage as it reduces the likelihood of people overhearing confidential conversations (*see* Question **15**). However, depending on the style of music chosen and the tastes of the listeners, it can also be an unwelcome distraction.

A children's area in the waiting room is always a good idea. If toys and playthings can be collected in one area with low tables and chairs for younger children, there is less likelihood of them disturbing other patients waiting. It is important that the toys and books are tidied regularly and that toys strewn about the floor do not present a hazard to people walking past.

▲ Question 37: Access for disabled people

We are currently revamping our surgery and wonder what we should take into account when making the premises as accessible as possible to disabled patients?

Many of the ways of ensuring accessibility seem obvious but are nonetheless often overlooked.

- Do you have street-level access at the main entrance? If not, can you provide a ramp for wheelchair users and for those with pushchairs?
- Are all the consulting rooms on the ground floor? If not, do you have a lift to upper floors that is large enough to take a wheelchair?
- Do you have large, clear notices on doors and in corridors to help partially sighted patients locate themselves within the building?
- Have you employed good lighting which will help people with poor vision?
- Is there good colour contrast on door handles and any switches so that those with defective sight can find their way around?
- Are lavatory doors clearly marked with visual symbols showing if they are suitable for male, female or disabled users? Are the ones designated for disabled users large enough for a wheelchair's turning circle? Are there handgrips on either side of the lavatory so that elderly or disabled patients can pull themselves to their feet?
- Are floor surfaces suitable for elderly or frail people to walk without slipping? And are the floor coverings appropriate for wheelchairs and pushchairs?
- A change in floor covering for corridors or pathways leading to the reception desk, for instance, will help blind patients to find their way to strategic points in the building.

There are a lot of things to think about when refurbishing premises. You cannot hope to incorporate every improvement that will make things easy for all kinds of patients but it is important that you try to include as many features as possible which will facilitate access for everyone, whatever their level of disability.

▲ Question 38: Facilities for mothers and babies

How important is it to provide nappy-changing facilities and baby-feeding areas for patients with babies?

With the increased pressures on general practice, most surgery buildings do not have sufficient space to provide all the services the GPs would wish. However, a small area adjacent to a washbasin in which mothers can safely change their babies does not take up much space and is much appreciated. A waist-high wide shelf (with a guard rail) on which a mother can place a baby in order to change its nappy is the ideal although most mothers would be happy just to have some privacy (preferably not on the floor of a public lavatory) in which to look after the baby's needs.

Babies can be fed in any room in which there is a comfortable chair and which is away from the main traffic of patients. This could be a staff common room or small interview room if you have such a thing but obviously you would have to ensure that any patient using such a room would not have access to confidential patient records or to other parts of the building that were out of bounds to patients.

The Department of Health encourages mothers to breastfeed their infants and each year issues the results of new research which claims to prove the positive health advantages throughout life to babies who have been breastfed for at least the first four months. New mothers often cite the non-availability of suitable facilities in public buildings to which they can withdraw to breastfeed their babies as a reason for electing to bottlefeed. Providers of health services, such as general practices, should perhaps be encouraging the practice of breastfeeding and should acknowledge such patients' needs for a little privacy in which to feed their babies and make available a small private room to which they can withdraw when necessary.

2

Information technology

As recently as ten years ago, there were few practices using computers. Some practices succumbed to the blandishments of suppliers of clinical systems who provided free equipment and software in return for access to anonymized patient data. However, the introduction of the new contract in 1990 prompted practices to consider computerization in order to maintain their age-sex register effectively and monitor target figures. Those practices that opted for fundholding had to expand their existing systems rapidly to incorporate the specialized packages required to control the financial transactions involved in the internal market. With prescribing budgets being increasingly squeezed by successive governments, GPs were being asked to prescribe more and more effectively and again computers helped this process.

The availability of data on the Internet in recent years has meant that doctors can gain up-to-date information from colleagues on clinical subjects at the press of a button. One note of caution should be sounded here. There is no effective mechanism for monitoring information on the Internet at the moment and so some of the data currently available are not always strictly accurate. This applies to information on medical matters as well as for wider issues.

The NHSNet which is planned for the NHS in the future will permit practices to link more effectively with each other, with hospital trusts, health authorities and pharmacies. Paperwork should be minimized and it is proposed that most data will be transferred electronically. More practices will take the opportunity of becoming, in effect, paperless. With fewer manual files, it will be increasingly important for practices to use computerized document management systems with standard protocols for secure storage and easy retrieval of patient data.

The change to primary care groups will necessitate networking practice and community staff computers together with local providers' systems to one main server. In Gloucestershire the cost of upgrading the hardware and providing this main server, the location of which has not yet been determined, is estimated to be about £3–5m. It is not clear just who will be expected to foot this bill.

Practice managers in general practice are taking on more responsibility for the financial management of the business and most now use spreadsheets and accounting software to monitor the financial position on a daily basis. The high cost of professional accountancy expertise means that practices will increasingly look to their managers to prepare the accounts each year, at least to trial balance, in order to try and reduce the accountant's fees.

Those practices which still farm out their payroll to an agency will almost certainly wish to rethink this and consider buying payroll software to enable the practice manager to do the payrun and thus save agency fees. Petty cash is unlikely to be still kept in a tin at the reception desk. Instead, a spreadsheet should be used to track cash spent on small items as well as to account for cash fees paid into the practice by patients. All fees will be recorded appropriately and banked regularly.

Few will need me to tell them that, as regards computerization in general practice, the goalposts are being moved constantly. Even during the few months spent researching this book, ideas regarding the computer requirements to facilitate primary care groups have changed dramatically, as have ideas for introducing the NHSNet to general practice. I have no reason to believe that such changes will stop or even slow down in the near future. It is becoming increasingly evident that if practices are to become more efficient and effective in the provision of health services to their patients, they will need to embrace technological change willingly rather than dragging their feet as some are still tempted to do.

▲ Question 39: Using computers effectively

Our practice has been computerized for several years now but the introduction of PCs to individual partners and to some of the staff was somewhat hit and miss. Data have been input in various ways and are often difficult to retrieve when we try to do a search. Any suggestions at this late stage as to how we can tidy things up?

Practices have been encouraged to computerize during recent years but few had any strategic plans for implementation of the equipment. This has meant that many practices have failed to produce protocols or guidelines for how information should be stored. If the information is stored randomly, using a wide variety of Read codes, then it is very difficult to use the computer for audit purposes which is one of the main advantages of the clinical system.

The first step is to get the partners to agree a set of guidelines. They will need to decide on just what information they want to store and how they want the relevant data input. They should agree which Read codes are to be used and then abide by these. Some systems can incorporate interactive protocols such as the SOPHIE system in Meditel or special templates in VAMP. This prompts the user to ask appropriate questions of the patient and enter relevant data in a pre-agreed format. This ensures standardization of data entry. Alternatively, staff can be given written protocols for entering data, for instance on how they should input pathology results, although these are increasingly being done automatically with pathology Links. This standardization of entry means that at a future date all the information can be pulled off the system by searching on agreed Read codes. For instance, an audit of all diabetic patients aged 50–75 who have taken a certain medication during the past six months would then be possible and meaningful.

Other areas where it is important to ensure that practice guidelines are followed closely is in the entering of details about newly registered patients. Practice income depends on accurate data being sent to the health authority. For instance, in practices where rural payments are made, it is important that the mileage is entered accurately so that the health authority will have the correct data on which to calculate such payments. These are based on the distance the patient lives from the surgery. When the practice is linked to the registration department, this should happen automatically but it is still wise to double-check that the correct mileages are registered at the health authority.

Information required for calculating eligibility for target payments is also crucial and so all immunizations should be entered using the agreed Read codes, to enable easy searching for those babies who have not yet had the required series of immunizations. For example, you can search on all five-year-olds who do not have a Read code for the diphtheria, tetanus and polio booster if staff have used the correct codes. Once identified, these children can then be caught opportunistically for their immunization, enabling the partners to reach the required targets of 90% of children in this age group fully immunized.

Using set protocols should ensure that all future information stored in the system is easily accessible. Altering past entries so that they conform is more difficult. However, if it is considered sufficiently important, a member of staff could search on a series of codes which might have been used in error to denote the same thing and could then alter them to the agreed coding for uniformity, if the system permits this. This will probably take some time but might be a worthwhile exercise for certain kinds of information, to which access in the future is likely to be important.

With the development of primary care groups and locality

purchasing, the requirements for set protocols and agreed standards will be even greater. If practices are going to be working in closer co-operation, it is obviously essential that they are all playing to the same rules.

▲ Question 40: Making best use of computers

We are aware that we do not use our system to its full capacity. Any suggestions on how we can make it work better for us?

Computers in general practice are often woefully underutilized. Initially, many GPs were content just to use the age-sex register and repeat-prescribing facility on the system. However, there are many ways in which information technology can be used to help in the management of the practice and treatment of patients.

For instance, a computer can be programed to remember how a GP prescribed previously and add this information to the picking list so that it is a simple matter to choose the same option. The system is not dictating how the GP prescribes but has 'learnt' their preferred way of prescribing and follows the pattern set. The system allows the GPs to highlight these personal prescribing patterns which can be useful when they get together for discussions on updating the practice formulary.

Electronic messaging can help reduce the stress on patients, GPs and staff caused by constant interruptions during consultations with urgent telephone calls from patients. Messages can be flashed on to the GP's consultation screen at any time and the message can be dealt with during a natural break in the consultation or between patients. Practices who have patients who regularly demand an urgent same-day appointment with a doctor can reassure them that the duty doctor will call them back shortly to discuss whether they really need to see a doctor immediately or whether an appointment with the practice nurse or with their own GP at a later date would be more appropriate.

The appointment program on most systems is a useful adjunct. It not only enables any person with access to a terminal and a telephone to make appointments but also offers other facilities such as auditing the numbers of patients seen by an individual GP, listing the persistent non-attenders and displaying the consulting history of a specific patient.

Macros are a useful way of speeding up repetitive tasks. A series of commands can be stored in a macro and it will then only be necessary to make one keystroke to achieve the desired task. Care has to be taken to ensure that the macros behave correctly but once set up properly, they can be used, for instance, to prescribe commonly used drugs. The dose, form, strength and quantity are all automatically determined taking into account the patient's age and other relevant factors. Another use for a macro might be in the storage of data in the patient's notes following a flu clinic. The macro might mark the notes, including information on the batch number of the inoculation, and also prepare details for submission to the PPA.

Practices are using the mail-merge facility to produce referral letters which incorporate all the required medical information and patient history which are automatically downloaded from the system. Desktop publishing software enables practices to produce their own stationery and leaflets (*see* Question **66**).

The question of audit was addressed in the first book in this series, entitled *Managing and Communicating*. For further information you should read *Making Sense of Audit*, details of which appear in the Further Reading list. Audit is a vital part of clinical and practice management and the computer is the ideal tool to facilitate the required searches.

Most practices now use computer software to keep a cashbook and produce spreadsheets to monitor the finances. To protect the confidentiality of the accounts and payroll, these can be run on a stand-alone PC in the manager's office.

Many GPs welcome the opportunity to load up-to-date clinical data on to their systems. Software which incorporates medical dictionaries or textbooks can be loaded on to the main system for use by all the clinicians and individual programs can be incorporated into the PCs of some of the partners for specialist use if required.

The uses of the practice computer would seem to be limitless. Access to the Internet and NHSNet is going to require a radical rethink by some practices. Just when they thought that they had a system large enough and fast enough to deal with their present and future needs, new applications have come along which will require further upgrading. This need to upgrade regularly is likely to continue, as in most businesses.

▲ Question 41: Upgrading hardware

Our system is slowing down appreciably as we install more PCs on to the network and load more and more data. It is obvious that we will have to upgrade the whole system shortly if it is not to grind to a halt. What points should we be considering?

The one rule that seems to be universally applicable is that whatever size and speed of computer you think you might require in the foreseeable future, you are sure to have underestimated. Computers have a built-in obsolescence and however you try to predict future needs, computer capacities and applications are increasing all the time and the one you thought would satisfy all your computer needs is out of date within a matter of years, if not months.

The first thing you should try to determine is how you plan to use the computer. Ask yourself some of the following questions.

- How many users do you envisage logging on at the same time? Is this likely to increase over time?
- How many peripherals are there at the moment and how many estimated in the future?

- What plans do you have to replace dumb terminals with PCs?
- Will all the partners be having a PC on their desk if they don't already?
- What about the practice nurses?
- What additional software is likely to be added?
- What does your contract with your main clinical supplier say about the acquisition of additional hardware?
- Do you put your maintenance contract at risk if you buy peripherals from other suppliers?

When deciding on which hardware to acquire, a possible first step would be to ask around other practices to see what they use and where they obtained their PCs and printers. You should not automatically assume that you will have to purchase from your original supplier. Although most practices are tied into agreements to purchase their main server from the supplier of their clinical system, you might be able to buy PCs or terminals more cheaply by mail order (although this is not recommended because of possible lack of support when problems occur) or from commercial retailers. Consulting experts at this stage is essential to avoid making an expensive mistake. Some suppliers of clinical systems charge fairly highly for the main server but provide additional hardware at reasonable prices in order not to alienate their customers. However, not all do, so it is worth shopping around.

Most practices are finding that PCs linked to the main server are gradually replacing dumb terminals because they are not much more expensive and are far more flexible. Even the kind of printers that those working in general practice require are becoming more sophisticated. As these items are replaced it is certainly worth doing some ringing around to get quotations for best prices. Some GPs have found that purchasing computer hardware via the Internet is a good option. Websites can show you the very latest deals, rather than articles in computer magazines which are often out of date by the time they are printed. The suppliers who advertise on the Internet also offer online support via E-mail.

▲ Question 42: Reuse of upgraded computer hardware

We are in the process of upgrading our seven-year-old computer hardware. Any suggestions as to what we can do with the old hardware?

The first rule of computing seems to be that all information technology becomes out of date very rapidly. You buy a system that offers more memory, faster speeds and greater capacity than your practice currently needs and within the space of a few years, or even months in some cases, it turns out to be inadequate for the new applications which the practice needs to install. It is, of course, often possible to upgrade existing hardware by incorporating additional memory but when this is no longer sufficient it will be necessary to buy a larger and faster machine.

However, old 286, 386 or 486 PCs need not be relegated to the scrapheap. They can be put to use in the practice running other software such as the accounts or payroll or as dedicated print or fax servers in networks; they can also be used to send E-mail internally. It is often useful to have the accounts on a separate PC in any case for reasons of confidentiality. Packages such as Quicken, Sage Moneywise, Microsoft Money or Maclean McNicoll GP accounting software can be installed on a smaller capacity computer for the sole use of the practice manager and lead partner. Likewise, access to the payroll can be restricted by installing it on a PC located in the practice manager's office and protected by password entry to which only she and the partners have access.

Old computers can also be used for desktop publishing. If you buy a relatively inexpensive desktop publishing package, you can save the practice money by using this to produce some of the practice stationery. For instance, you can design headed paper and compliment slips with the practice logo and this can be produced in full colour, using several colours in the one design for little additional cost. You can also personalize the headed paper for individual GPs and even amend it simply when a partner retires or leaves the practice (*see* Question **66**).

The practice booklet can be produced in the surgery and you can design your own information leaflets all using smaller capacity computers which are no longer large enough to cope with the clinical system and networking requirements. So the old equipment will not be wasted; there are plenty of uses to which it can be put.

▲ Question 43: PCs in consulting rooms

The doctors in our practice are reluctant to have computers in their consulting rooms because they fear that the presence of the monitor on their desk will hinder good interaction with the patient. What particular advantages can I stress in order to persuade them to have a PC to hand during a consultation?

This is a common problem. However, those GPs who have accepted a screen on their desks have found that patients actually appreciate the fact that the doctor has all their details at his fingertips without having to fumble through wads of medical records stuffed into a bulging Lloyd George envelope. Some GPs have installed medical textbook software such as Bodyworks or E-BNF onto their systems and the graphic displays of parts of the human body and the effect of various ailments have proved popular with some patients. Patients are often intrigued to see illustrated on the screen what the GP is trying to explain to them verbally about their particular condition.

The GP can use the screen prompts to remind patients about overdue prescriptions, cytology recall or the need for a diabetic check-up. The GP can also be prompted to offer contraceptive advice or a tetanus booster. All these things will almost certainly be considered as a benefit by the patient rather than as an intrusion.

If the practice has a computerized appointment system, the doctors can see at a glance the list of their patients for each surgery. Some would claim that it is sometimes better not to know when heartsink patients are booked but again the advantages of being able to prepare for what lies ahead have to be weighed against any forebodings felt. Clinicians can book a follow-up appointment with patients while they are still sitting with them.

Another great asset with some systems is that urgent messages for the doctor can be flashed onto the consulting screen by a member of staff, without the need to interrupt the consultation by telephoning. This facility has been welcomed by staff, doctors and patients alike as it can certainly reduce the stress which constant audible interruptions can cause (*see* Question **65** on electronic messaging).

If the doctors believe that the computer will get in the way of the consultation, the actual monitor can be placed to one side of the desk so that it does not come between patient and doctor. If the GP prefers not to enter notes in the presence of the patient, he can always add details after the patient has left and before he calls the next one. The doctors will of course have to be very careful to clear each patient's data from the screen following each consultation to ensure confidentiality.

Some doctors prefer to dictate referral letters in the presence of the patient. Using voice-operated software, the GP could even dictate straight onto the computer during the consultation so that the patient can be confident that the referral has indeed been made. However, the technology for this is still in its infancy and it might be wise to wait until the software has been further refined before making a decision to acquire it.

▲ Question 44: Laptops versus palmtops

We are considering buying a laptop computer for the duty doctor to take when making calls. Would a smaller palmtop be more suitable?

Palmtop computers are generally about one-third of the size of laptops, and weigh only 800 g as opposed to the 2.5 kg that a laptop is likely to weigh. A palmtop will have a greater battery life (approximately ten times as long) and is now available with a colour screen. Palmtops boot up instantly at the press of a button since the operating systems and applications are stored in ROM. Both palmtops and laptops come with the usual software for word processing and spreadsheets, database handling and record access via modem. Both the laptop and the palmtop can be connected by cable directly to a PC and the information shared in a form of network.

The keyboard on the palmtop is difficult to use for someone who touch types but for accessing data it is adequate. The laptop has a mouse and a full-size keyboard. Currently, laptops are about twice the price of palmtops, with prices starting at about £1000, but they can be more depending on their level of sophistication.

If portability is the main issue, then obviously the palmtop will win as it is far more compact and would fit easily into a doctor's bag. However, the greater versatility of the laptop has meant that many GPs have chosen this option for use by the doctor on call.

▲ Question 45: Change to new supplier

We are becoming increasingly dissatisfied with our clinical system which we have had since the days when suppliers were giving computer hardware and software freely to GPs in return for clinical data on patients obtained from the system. We are considering switching to another system. What points should we be looking for when making our decision?

Conversion to a new system is not a step to be taken lightly as there are obvious risks associated with transferring clinical data, not least of which is the real fear of losing some of the data – particularly linked items – in the transmission process. It is also wise to check whether changes to software will be necessary when primary care groups become better established and all practices in the group are linked in a local network, as seems to be the DoH's intention. It is planned that health authorities will have to allocate part of their budget to updating GP systems and software yet again and it is likely that the practices will not be expected to pay for such upgrading themselves. This is another good reason for contacting your health authority before you decide to change your software.

That said, you are not alone if you really are dissatisfied with the service your present supplier is offering and they supply you both with software and hardware. More and more practices are making the decision to switch because of uncertainty about reaccreditation and the future viability of certain GP computer companies. Some pundits are predicting that in the next five to ten years, only about three suppliers of clinical systems for use in general practice will remain. The others will either have fallen by the wayside or been taken over by one of the larger companies.

Practices are also preparing to change the way they use their system in the present climate of general practice, with the ultimate goal of becoming a paperless practice. Electronic transmission of data between all the various agencies linked to primary care means that not only will systems have to become more sophisticated but also they will need to be able to network effectively. Many GPs feel that their present system is unlikely to be able to cope with the increasing amount of data that they might wish to store and transfer electronically in the future.

However, once you have taken this into account and the partners decide that they should proceed with a change of supplier, your first step should be to ask around among other local practices to discover which systems they use and whether they are satisfied with them. You should be asking the partners and staff what they plan to do with the new system.

- Is the intention to store more complex data?
- Do they want to make better use of clinical audit?
- Does the system you are considering have the capability to perform the searches you will require?
- How will the government requirements for increasing computer links with primary care groups, hospitals and health authorities be handled by your proposed new system?

When you have decided on some alternative suppliers that you think might serve your needs, you should contact one or two practices who have switched from the same supplier that you have to the proposed one. The supplier of the new system should be able to provide the names of such customers but you should be aware that they are unlikely to put you in contact with dissatisfied clients! It is particularly important that the switch between systems has been made in the same way as you intend because changes from other systems are inevitably different, although not necessarily beset by any fewer problems.

You will need to know just which areas caused the most problems. For instance, many practices have found that repeat-prescribing information has been distorted in the transmission to a new system. Others have found that recalls for cytology or immunizations have been affected. You should make sure that any such problems which occur as a result of the conversion are mitigated as far as possible and that you have contingency plans for a worst-case scenario of lost or distorted data. Adequate verified back-ups will be essential in case you have to restore data from the previous system.

You will need a small group – lead GP partner, practice manager and computer manager, perhaps – to oversee the installation of the new system. You will also need to have in place a schedule for training GPs, nurses and staff in the use of the new software. It is vital that everyone follows set protocols for the entering of data with agreed codes. Audit depends on good searches and these are only possible if relevant codes are used consistently by everyone.

The installation itself can be time consuming and recabling can be a nightmare if it takes place during the working day. Try to obtain quotes from companies who are prepared to work at weekends in order to install the cabling in the shortest possible period and with the least disruption to the staff and patients.

Other questions you should be asking are:

- Who is going to be responsible for the process of transferring the data from start to finish?
- How long between the date the new supplier takes a copy of the data and the actual upgrade? (It can sometimes be up to a month before you can add new data to the system.)
- Who is going to take charge of the day-to-day implementation?
- Is there a computer manager or partner within the practice who will take on the training of others in the team?
- Who will write the protocols which will determine how information is added to the system?
- Does the new supplier guarantee that essential data will not be lost in the transfer?

Some practices have found that leaving the old system running on a separate PC, at least for a few months, can be invaluable for accessing data that may have been damaged during conversion. Speaking to several practices that have recently undergone a conversion, all of them say that if you accept that anything that can go wrong will go wrong, you will be well prepared.

▲ Question 46: Computer maintenance contracts

Do we have to have contracts covering the maintenance on all our computer hardware? Our supplier insists on our purchasing all our hardware, as well as the medical system, from them and this can mean very high maintenance costs.

Computer maintenance contracts are supposed to bring peace of mind, but often they become an expensive nightmare. It is absolutely essential that you have a maintenance contract for your main server and perhaps the more expensive and essential printers. However, it is generally acknowledged that practices do not need to take out service agreements on all the peripheral hardware in the practice. Individual PCs, dumb terminals, keyboards and many of the printers do not need to be covered after the initial warranty lapses. For instance, it is usually considered to be more cost effective to replace an occasional faulty terminal (one of perhaps ten or 15 in the practice) rather than have an expensive maintenance agreement covering the whole lot.

Some practices keep spare equipment to replace any items that break down. Some printers and PCs can also be cheaper to replace as needed rather than maintaining them regularly for years. The maintenance contract usually only covers repair when something goes wrong rather than any regular servicing. As the life of most computer hardware is seldom more than a few years before it becomes obsolete, it would seem sensible to consider very carefully just which items you need to cover.

It is not always necessary to purchase all your hardware through your main supplier. However, if you use an alternative supplier you will need to make sure that there is no debate about responsibility when something goes wrong. Suppliers are all too eager to claim that the problem lies in the hardware (bought elsewhere) rather than in their software or linked hardware. Increasingly practices are buying PCs and printers much more cheaply by mail order or on the high street and once the warranty expires, are just trusting to luck or taking out separate, and usually less expensive, cover.

▲ Question 47: Technical support/back-up

The supplier of our main clinical system is proving less and less accessible. We ring for 20 or 30 minutes at a time without getting a reply. Their staff do not seem able to sort out problems easily over the telephone any more. Sometimes we are passed from person to person and still no one seems to know the solution. Is there any way in which we can obtain a better service than this?

Some suppliers have found it difficult to keep up with the rapid expansion in the number of GP customers that has taken place over recent years. Companies are finding it difficult to attract and retain well-trained staff who are able to solve problems encountered by relatively inexperienced users of the system.

Some practices have decided to switch systems (*see* Question 45), transferring all their data to a new system in the hope that the new company will provide a more efficient technical support service. If you do decide this might be an option for your practice, you should research the matter carefully before taking the plunge because switching can sometimes produce more problems than it solves. You will need to talk to other practices who have transferred from the same system and to the same new supplier that you are contemplating. The company will be pleased to give you names of satisfied customers.

If you elect to remain with the same company but wish them to improve their support, you can try writing to the senior executive of the firm stating your specific complaints. It is helpful if you can quote dates and times and particular instances of undue delay in problem solving. This is when a computer log becomes invaluable.

In it should be kept details of all problems experienced with either software or hardware. Dates should be noted and details of the solution ultimately found and who provided it. It is also useful to note how long telephone calls to helpdesks lasted in specific instances. It is far more effective to say to the managing director of your supplier that your staff called three times during one day and on each occasion had to wait in excess of 30 minutes for a response rather than just informing him that his helpline is inaccessible.

You can also ask among your local user group for details of problems they have experienced with the same clinical system supplier. If you do not belong to a local user group, it might be worth considering joining or forming one in order to provide more clout when approaching the supplier. If a group of unhappy customers contact them *en masse*, they are more likely to sit up and take notice of your complaints.

If you continue to receive poor service well below the standard promised by the supplier, as a last resort you can always state your intention of withholding maintenance payments until matters are rectified to your satisfaction. You should take care when using this sanction, however, and read the small print in your contract with the company before taking any direct action.

▲ Question 48: IT manager

We have the usual collection of complicated computer technology in our practice and no one seems to understand how it works. Whenever anything goes wrong, we have to call the suppliers of our clinical system who also provided most of the hardware and they are not always readily available to help when we need them. What can we do to improve matters?

Most practices are now computerized but many are unable to use their expensive systems to full advantage because no one in the practice appreciates or understands the full potential of the system. In addition, users are not trained in how to input data accurately or access information readily. Problems inevitably occur which require specialized help to disentangle them.

One of the answers might be to appoint one of the existing staff with a particular interest in computers to be the computer manager. This might even be you yourself or alternatively one of the partners might want to take on the role. If one of the GPs does decide to manage the IT within the practice, the other partners might consider employing a locum to cover a half session a week to enable him to have protected time in which to problem solve. However, it is not an ideal solution since inevitably the doctor will not be available for crisis management most of the time and this is one of the main roles that the IT manager should be expected to take.

Alternatively, you might decide to recruit someone new to the practice – not necessarily full time – to fulfil this role. Whoever is designated as computer manager will almost certainly need to undergo regular training not only in the medical software but also in the basics of hardware maintenance. For instance, most practices have many different kinds of printers from the laserjet in the secretary's office to the inkjets or dot matrix printers in the GPs' consulting rooms. Specialized knowledge will be required to fix problems on most of the hardware. Having a member of staff who can put right minor hardware problems can save a great deal of time and hassle for the rest of the users.

In addition to the clinical software, there will also be various other programs in use such as the payroll and accounting packages. There are usually helplines associated with this software but the helpdesk staff are not always readily available when you need their services. If the IT manager can sort out most of the more trivial problems, any expense involved in training them should prove an excellent investment in time and money.

▲ Question 49: Training

Few of our staff have been given proper training in how to use computers in general and our medical system in particular. As a result, information is input in a variety of ways which makes it difficult to search the system for information. What is the best way of remedying this situation?

IT training in general practice is one of the most neglected aspects of GP computing. It is vital that staff (and doctors) know how to use the system effectively. Many practices have set protocols which are followed by anyone inputting clinical data such as laboratory test results, cytology recalls, contraception claims or details of immunizations. These protocols should be written down, agreed by the partners and then distributed to all members of staff who will be inputting such data. Links also necessitates inputting in an agreed format in order to ensure standardized data entries.

If staff are inconsistent in their use of codes, it might be worthwhile having a group training session to stress the importance of adhering to the agreed protocols and explaining why using a variety of codes for the same information can cause problems when searches are being made. It is also important that information appears on the correct 'screen' so that it is instantly available to clinicians when patients consult them.

It is helpful if new staff, including nurses, receptionists, secretaries and even locum GPs, have training sessions in the use of the practice computer as part of their induction program. Such training sessions can be spread over a period of time so that the individual is able to absorb the information and put it into practice before embarking on the next phase of learning. If you have a computer manager (*see* Question **48**) then it should be incumbent upon them to arrange regular training courses for the staff and this aspect of their job should be written into their contract.

Too many computer systems were introduced on an ad hoc basis in the past without much thought as to how they would be used.

As a result, much of the information has been stored in an inconsistent and random way which renders audit almost impossible. As more and more practices move towards the ideal of a paperless system, with patient data transmitted electronically between health authority, trust, pharmacy and practice, it is vital that this information is stored in an easily accessible and universally acceptable form.

▲ Question 50: Health and safety issues associated with using VDUs

What are the health and safety regulations regarding the use of VDUs? I understand that as employers, the GPs have an obligation to any staff using computers to make sure they are not harmed by constant use of the machines.

Visual display units (VDUs) feature increasingly in general practice and most members of staff now use them during their working day at some time. Health problems often associated with the use of computers are not caused directly by the VDUs themselves but are more likely to result from the way in which they are used. The Health and Safety (Display Screen Equipment) Regulations 1992 are the rules governing use of VDUs.

Basically, these regulations do not contain detailed technical specifications but instead set general objectives. Employers are required to look at individual workstations and their users in order to assess and endeavour to reduce the likely risks associated with long-term use of the computers. Things to look for include ensuring that all VDUs have an adjustable brightness and contrast control for the screen so that individuals can adjust these to suit the particular task. All staff working at computers should take regular short breaks in order to avoid straining their eyes or sitting in the same position for long periods. Staff are entitled to ask their employer to pay for an eyesight test. Staff should be trained in how to use the workstation equipment safely which will include simple things like adjusting the height of the chair to avoid excessive strain or moving the VDU away from the window to avoid light reflections on the screen.

If you are in any doubt about what measures you should be taking to ensure the health of personnel using computers, then you can obtain a copy of the relevant regulations from the Health and Safety Executive (HSE Books) whose address is given at the end of this book.

▲ Question 51: Patient confidentiality

The government seems set on improving electronic links between practices and the wider NHS network. I am concerned that patient confidentiality may be breached during the electronic transmission of data between hospital trusts, health authorities and ourselves. What provision is being made to prevent any such breach?

Computer links between practices and other agencies involved in primary health care are set to increase dramatically in the near future. In order to safeguard confidentiality in the electronic transmission of patient data, the proposal is that the patients' ten-digit NHS number will be used in all transfers and this will offer the only individual identification on any information. There will be no names or other identifiable information such as addresses or postcodes used during the transmission of such data. Using only the NHS number should mean that confidentiality is assured.

However, a more easily overlooked possible breach of confidentiality can occur within the practice, when a clinician leaves the previous patient's details clearly visible on the computer screen after the next patient has entered the consulting room. This is particularly unfortunate if the clinician is called away briefly to an emergency elsewhere and the patient has the opportunity to read the details unobserved. Such breaches occur regularly and I know of cases where it has been particularly damaging. All doctors and staff should be reminded of the danger of allowing such a breach to occur and should take steps to guard against it.

The reception desk is another place where the VDU has to be carefully screened from public gaze. Sometimes placing a mesh guard over the screen can make it impossible to see from the patient's angle of view, as well as helping to reduce glare reflecting into the eyes of the user.

Use of passwords to access sensitive data is also essential (*see* Question **52**). Most clinical systems have 'hidden' screens on which highly confidential data can be stored and accessed only by the relevant clinician. For instance, details of HIV status or the results of an AIDS test might be stored in this way to prevent access by anyone else.

It is important to guard against any possible breach of confidentiality in whatever form and with computer data it is particularly important to review procedures regularly to ensure that no such breach can occur. The practice should be on the Data Protection Register if it stores data electronically and this registration needs to be renewed regularly. You should make yourself aware of the obligations this registration imposes with regard to protecting the confidentiality of all patient data held on your system. The address of the Data Protection Agency is given at the end of the book.

▲ Question 52: User identification and passwords

We have a problem identifying which member of staff has input certain data onto the practice computer system. The initials of a member of the team appear beside the particular entry but it does not always relate to the individual who made the entry. Any suggestions as to how we can ensure consistency?

The reason for this is almost certainly that the staff are failing to log out of an individual terminal or PC when they finish working. This means that the next person to use that particular screen will continue adding data but will not have logged in individually and so all information will be attributed to the previous user.

A strict rule should be adhered to whereby staff are given an individual password and ID and are required to use these when they input any data. They should log off from the system every time they leave their desk unattended for any length of time. Likewise, any member of staff starting work at a computer should make sure that they log out and log in again if the system is not already back to the prompt for a password.

Passwords should be confidential and doctors and staff should be encouraged to change theirs regularly, at least several times a year. In my experience few users bother to do this but it is a necessary part of ensuring access is strictly limited. It is perhaps an obvious point but worth mentioning that users should choose a word for their password that is easy to remember and difficult to guess. The name of their oft-mentioned spouse or pet dog is unlikely to fall into this category. With the increase in computer networking set to happen in the near future with the onset of primary care groups, it is particularly important to guard against the possibility of outsiders hacking into the system.

▲ Question 53: The Internet/Intranet

I keep hearing about the Intranet in relation to the NHS and wonder how this differs from the Internet and World Wide Web mentioned in the media.

The Internet is a worldwide network of computers, from large mainframes to smaller individual PCs, linked in the main by telephone lines. For GPs the Internet offers the chance to communicate with people across the world on matters of common interest but there are also educational packages on the World Wide Web of specific relevance to doctors and other clinicians. Access to the Internet allows GPs to liaise with others in order to air clinical problems or seek information on medical matters.

There are many Internet service providers (ISPs) in the UK and some are easier to use than others. If you decide to link up to the Internet, you should shop around for a service provider who offers the kind of access you will require. Most ISPs will offer you a month's free trial access (but will usually require your credit card number in the first instance). Do check that access to the ISP you choose is by way of a *local* telephone call to keep costs down. Also, it is important to check that the company has sufficient modems at their end to take calls from its many users at busy times. You will require an integral web browser, an E-mail program and a simple scheduling facility which automates the sending and receiving of mail. Most of those GPs who have gone online find that they use the Internet for three main purposes:

- as an information resource
- for E-mail
- for obtaining computer files and programs.

As more and more users come online, the World Wide Web's value will increase and Internet contact between practices will become commonplace. The mutual support and exchange of ideas can be invaluable for busy professionals. GPs can swap notes about clinical and administrative problems with colleagues in other practices.

In order to have access to the Internet, the practice will need a computer with a modem, a telephone line and special software from an ISP as discussed above. The computer will need to be at least a Pentium 75 with 16 Mb RAM and a modem of 28 800 bps as a minimum. The higher the number of kilobytes per second that the modem can transmit, the faster you will receive information from the World Wide Web. Some practices have tried with a slower computer but have found that their telephone bills were correspondingly higher. It can also be frustrating having to wait interminably for information to come up on the screen.

Once you have become familiar with logging on to the Internet, you might perhaps want to create your own website. A website holds information which is controlled (and updated) by you and is accessible to other users.

A few tips on accessing the Internet from experienced GP users include the following.

- Consult computer magazines as well as colleagues working in other practices when choosing online servers as costs can vary greatly.
- Fast modems are mainly an advantage if your computer is powerful enough to make use of the speed.
- Do not send confidential information via E-mail as it is not secure.
- Invest in antivirus software before you start using the Internet.
- Avoid using a computer holding patient details when accessing the Internet as a persistent hacker might gain entry to your system.

An Intranet, on the other hand, could be a number of PCs linked between GP surgeries, health authorities, pharmacies and hospital trusts in a local area network with a web server. The government is promoting the NHSNet (a form of Intranet) as the way forward for the NHS. All the users would have a browser to view applications and many users of Intranets can also access the Internet. It makes sense that the vast investment in computerization in all the different sectors should be put to good use linking all together. Currently there is a problem with rationalizing the different systems installed in the various practices and trusts but eventually it is hoped that a standard will be obtained to allow all to communicate. Already patient information is being transmitted via modem directly to the computer system at the other end which means that pathology results, patient registration data and discharge letters can all be passed quickly and efficiently via the system without a member of staff having to input the information at either end. However, an Intranet will permit great networking. The question of patient confidentiality will be addressed by using just the NHS number for patient identification.

▲ Question 54: E-mail

How might e-mail be of use in our practice? We are wondering whether to link up to the Internet but feel it might be an expensive option unless we can make use of all the facilities.

E-mail is a cheap and simple way to send messages for the price of a single telephone call. It is an efficient and cost-effective way of sending information speedily and when you have it, you will wonder how you made do with just a fax machine. The one main problem is that, of course, not everyone that you might wish to contact will have an e-mail address. However, general practices are increasingly going online and so the possibilities for networking among GPs and practice managers are immense.

Networking has always been important for practice managers who can find themselves very isolated in their individual practices. Networking via the computer will be a most welcome way of keeping in touch with other practices and discovering joint solutions to common problems. It is likely to be particularly popular with far-flung practices as it will enable them to communicate immediately with others a long distance away but who might well be experiencing similar problems. There can be no question of a conflict of interest or of competitive advantage where practices many miles apart choose to share information.

▲ Question 55: NHSNet

I have seen mention of the NHSNet in the recent White Paper. Just what does this mean and how is it likely to affect those of us working in general practice?

The White Paper published in December 1997 proposed yet more changes for computerization in the NHS, with a view to linking secondary and primary care services via the NHSNet, a network of computer systems in the health sector. The plan is for most information to be transferred electronically, often in formatted order so as to speed up transmission. The introduction of this system is set to be completed by the year 2002 and so there are likely to be many changes in the next few years as everyone working in the NHS moves towards this goal.

The DoH recognized that with the introduction of fundholding, computerization in general practice was geared very much to 'supporting the transaction processes of the internal market'. In the recent White Paper they state their belief that 'This has been at the expense of realizing the potential of IT to support front-line staff in delivering benefits to patients'. They are now determined to 'harness the enormous potential benefits of IT to support the drive for quality and efficiency in the NHS'.

They aim to do this by making patient records electronically available when they are required, if at all possible. By using the NHSNet linking general practice computers to those in health authorities, hospital trusts and pharmacies, the plan is to bring patients not only faster test results but also online booking of appointments for outpatient appointments and up-to-date specialist advice.

The Internet is currently expanding at a phenomenal rate and the hope is that this will also be used to provide the public with knowledge about health, illness and which treatments are currently considered best practice.

The DoH also plan to develop telemedicine to ensure specialist skills are available even in the most inaccessible parts of the country. The department is determined to attempt the creation of seamless computer communication between all the NHS agencies involved in providing services to patients.

▲ Question 56: Modems

Can you explain a little about what we should look for when choosing a modem so that we can send faxes and ultimately access the Internet?

The speed of the modem is the all-important factor in choosing which one will best suit you. However, you should bear in mind that sending faxes via the modem will not necessarily be faster because the speed of transmission will be dependent on the speed of the receiving fax machine, which may still be relatively slow.

The new standard (as I write at the beginning of 1998) is the K56 which is basically a 56 000 bps modem that uses special software to receive data at twice the normal rate. Some models include facilities such as CD-ROM, enabling connection to the major Internet providers. The modem is supported by the Windows 95 driver which means that its compatibility with the standard Windows programs is assured. In theory, the speed of this modem should mean that you spend less time on the Internet since it should access your chosen websites faster. However, in practice this may not be apparent.

If you merely want to send faxes it is probably not worthwhile buying to the K56 standard; a 33 600 bps would be sufficient. However, if you want to be sure that you can access the Internet easily in the future, then it is essential to go for the faster modem.

Installation of the modem is relatively simple but you need to open the computer and insert the modem card in a vacant slot. It is obviously wise to have someone who knows what they are doing to access the computer in this way and if you are in any doubt about your ability to do it successfully, I would advocate calling in an expert.

▲ Question 57: Repeat prescribing

When we first acquired our practice computer almost ten years ago we mainly used it for the age-sex register and for repeat prescribing. Is there any way that we can use all this information on medication that we have accumulated?

Many practices found that their computer was ideal for relieving doctors and staff of the chore of writing repeat prescriptions for patients. Over the years a great deal of data is now stored on patterns of prescribing medication. It should be possible to target specific types of patient and audit medication usage. One of the joys of having information on computer is that it should be possible to search on certain codes in order to derive statistical information which can be used in the clinical management of prescribing.

GPs are being encouraged by the DoH to examine their prescribing and see if they can find ways of reducing some of the vast medication costs that the NHS pays each year. Generic prescribing has been one way in which costs have been cut over recent years as a result of various government initiatives to persuade GPs to prescribe cost effectively. In addition, GPs and pharmacist advisers have been able to identify certain areas where branded drugs can prove cheaper if only because they are more effective in specific circumstances and require fewer doses to achieve the desired result.

If in any doubt on how to go about auditing the GPs' prescribing patterns, you should consult your pharmacist adviser at the health authority. The partners might also need to obtain copies of recent third-level PACT data for each GP.

One other point on prescriptions. Nottingham Trent University is developing technology which will recognize handwritten scripts and convert them into print.

The GP could write on a palmtop computer and the prescription would be filed into the patient's record or printed out at the press of a button. It is anticipated that the system will be commercially available in three or four years' time.

▲ Question 58: Prodigy – prescribing support software

I heard one of the GPs mention some computer software called Prodigy. What does this stand for?

The name Prodigy is formed from the words '**P**rescribing **RatiOn**ally with **D**ecision support **In** **G**eneral practice stud**Y**'. It is a computerized prescribing aid which was piloted by 137 GPs in 1996. Further evaluation took place during 1997. The aim of the software is to help reduce the NHS prescribing budget by £1.5 billion and with this in mind the system has been set up to recommend the three most cost-effective drugs for a given diagnosis. It is anticipated that Prodigy will be rolled out gradually during 1998 and use of the system will be voluntary.

A competing system, Capsule, is being developed by the Imperial Cancer Research Fund for use by GPs. This takes into account the patient's history and current medication and provides patient-specific advice and helps to prevent adverse drug interactions. In initial studies the system significantly increased generic prescribing which helped to reduce costs. However, occasionally the GP would be prompted to prescribe a more expensive branded mediation simply because it was more effective and, in the long run, might even prove to be cheaper. The main aim is to promote rational prescribing. In pilots it was found that GPs preferred the

Capsule system because it gave patient-specific advice and reasons for the drug recommendations.

In the meantime some practices are piloting the PACTline system which will enable a hospital, for instance, to interrogate an individual patient's notes electronically to see whether the patient is allergic to penicillin. The GPs will be able to access PACT data electronically not only for their own practice but also for national and county prescribing percentages.

▲ Question 59: Scanner

Our practice is considering buying a scanner with which to scan consultant letters and other patient records into our system. How effective are they and what should we be considering when deciding on which one to buy?

Scanners are improving all the time and by the time you read this, scanner technology may well have advanced further. Practices trying to reduce the amount of paper they have to store are increasingly storing data in electronic form. In order to do this, rather than key in lengthy letters and reports, they use a scanner to transfer information from a consultant's letter or discharge summary, for example, onto the patient's computer notes. At the time of writing in early 1998 many practices are using registration and items-of-service Links to exchange specific information with their health authority. However, the kind of data that can be transferred is currently rather limited.

If the practice does decide to buy a scanner, some of the points which should be considered include:

- *the optical resolution* – the sharpness of the image the scanner can produce. Figures of 300 dots per inch (dpi) are sufficient for text but 600 dpi are considered to be the minimum necessary for clear photographic images

- *automatic document feed* – this might cost as much as the scanner itself but if you plan to feed in piles of letters and information it can easily repay you in staff time saved in feeding documents individually
- *the correct port* – check that your computer has the right kind of port to suit the chosen scanner. Some require a parallel port, others an SCSI or serial port
- *graphics packages* – many scanners come with a free 'bundled' graphics package such as Photoshop or Photopaint. This type of software enables you to manipulate the size, colour and shape of the photographic images.

Most scanners are in the price range of £150 to £800 but there are more expensive (and more complex) ones available. As with most technology, prices are falling all the time as models are superseded and bigger (or smaller!) and better ones introduced.

One last thought. In the White Paper published in December 1997, the government set a goal of all practices having computer systems which will allow them to link with hospitals and the health authority by the year 2002. With the likely improvements in computer networking (the NHSNet) you might find that the need to scan in documents diminishes as more information is transmitted electronically between hospitals, health authorities and practices. It will certainly serve to reduce the need for scanning although it is unlikely to do away with the need altogether. However, it might be wise to bear all this in mind when considering whether a scanner is really essential at this stage.

▲ Question 60: Voice-operated software

One of the GPs wants his partners to agree to buy a voice-operated computer to enable him to dictate his own referral letters. Is this a good idea?

Voice-operated software, such as the IBM Voicetype, has improved dramatically over recent months. The latest version of the IBM software is called 'Simply Speaking'. Dragon, an American company, produce a voice-activated system called 'Dictate' which has a British English version called 'Personal Addition'. Microsoft have their 'Naturally Speaking Solo' software which does much the same thing.

To install the software you will require a Pentium with a minimum of 48 Mb RAM. The installation will take some time as the computer has to be taught to recognize an individual voice and pronunciation. Even when you have done the introductory work involved in customizing the system to your voice, you will still have to input the health dictionary as the software will probably come with only the normal standard commercial vocabulary. The dictator will need to wear a headset in order to dictate.

Once the medical dictionary has been loaded and you have acclimatized the system to your voice, you should be able to achieve about 90% accuracy fairly swiftly and this standard will be improved upon as you continue to dictate and correct errors in the computer's interpretation of your dictation. Be prepared for some hilarious mistakes in the first instance. One clergyman friend of mine trying to dictate a sermon found that 'Mount Sinai' appeared as 'melt cyanide' and he gave up after trying 'Let no flocks or herds feed' which even at a second attempt came out as 'let no clocks or birds seed'. And you should realize that if you try to dictate while you have a cold, the system will have even greater trouble in understanding and interpreting the dictation correctly.

You should warn the doctor that it is unlikely that he will ever want to undertake the whole process of producing his own referral letters, however proficient he becomes at using the system. Formatting the document, addressing and printing envelopes can be time consuming for those not used to word processing and even for those who are. Other GPs have found that they can dictate the required text and insert it into a skeleton letter on the main system for their secretary to address and present for signature. It can also be used to produce articles and reports but again it is probably less time consuming to have a secretary produce the final draft.

Using such a voice recognition system does require a fair amount of computer memory if it is to work well. Some doctors report having had several crashes caused by dictation overruns because they had insufficient RAM.

▲ Question 61: GP Links

I manage a small single-partner practice and we have only recently become computerized. We are in the process of linking up with the health authority for registration Links. Are there any tips you can give me so that we avoid some of the possible pitfalls in this linking?

As with most changes in computer usage, the most important part of the process is to ensure that adequate preparation takes place. Many practices have found that they require additional staff to cope with the workload involved in running GP Links, particularly when they move on to item-of-service claiming. Ongoing training for staff involved in maintaining the Links and inputting the data is essential. However, you will first need to rationalize your patient list with that of the health authority prior to linking. It is obviously essential that you have the names and addresses of your patients exactly the same in every detail. In the past practices have found this process very revealing and somewhat dispiriting as ghost patients have appeared on the system, having lurked there for years long after moving away and registering elsewhere.

Once you have established that your lists are identical, you will then need to meet with the member of the health authority staff in charge of linking in order to discuss the exact process of how and when the data will be transmitted and the date when the practice link is expected to go 'live'.

When the system is up and running, the data will be sent down the line at the end of each day and receptionists will find that the amount of paperwork they are required to do when registering a patient will diminish rapidly. Once you have incorporated registration Links into your practice system, you will then perhaps be ready to consider items-of-service Links which provides another way of saving on paperwork when making the claims. You should be aware of any cut-off dates for items-of-service claims after which data cannot be added to the system while the HA brings their information in line and up to date.

One last point needs to be stressed. Once you have Links established and running well, do not imagine that you can cease checking claims and registrations. There is still scope for human error in the acceptance of data at the health authority end. For instance, some practices have found that their child health surveillance claims and rural practice payments have not been paid in full because of an administrative glitch in the system. The data were sent correctly but for some reason they were not accepted on to the health authority system and no note of this rejection was given to the practice. Ongoing monitoring and regular audit of all fees paid by the health authority are therefore essential.

▲ Question 62: Computerized accounts

I took up my appointment as practice manager in a small city centre practice recently and was appalled to discover that the senior partner was 'doing the books' by the simple expedient of writing down figures in a ledger from the bank statement when it arrived. I would like to set up a proper cashbook and would like to know if I should do this manually or whether there are good computer packages available specifically for use in general practice.

You are not alone in having a practice where one of the partners still insists on doing the books, even though it sounds as if he, like most busy GPs, has little time in which to do it properly. I came across one practice recently where no accounts were kept at all and the proverbial brown paper bag and shoe boxes containing all the invoices and remittances were delivered to the accountants at the year end for sorting out. This is obviously a very expensive option for preparing the accounts. The accountants charge by the amount of time they spend preparing the accounts and at £100+ per hour it can prove very costly not to do the basic book keeping in the practice. If all the day-to-day entries are made in the cashbook and regular bank reconciliations are undertaken, then the time the accountants take to produce the accounts will be appreciably less and the cost correspondingly reduced. (Managing the practice finances is discussed fully in *Finance and Administration*, the second book in the Practice Manager Library series.)

There are several commercial accounting and cashbook software packages available such as Quicken, Microsoft Money v.4 and Sage Moneywise that are used by many GPs in their practices. MS Money is only available if you have Windows 95. With these systems bank reconciliations can be done regularly, enabling you to monitor the bank balances. However, the systems allow for the basic cashbook but not, of course, a health authority ledger as they are not geared specifically to general practice finances – which are idiosyncratic to say the least.

The Maclean McNicoll GP accounts system, on the other hand, is specifically written for GPs and includes not only a cashbook for all income and expenditure entries but also a special ledger which permits year-on-year comparison of quarterly statement payments. There is a facility to include health authority figures and Medeconomics national average figures for comparison. Analysis can be done on any section of the accounts and details of previous years' figures are archived on the system and can be drawn on for comparison. It is very simple to operate and once set up with the appropriate analysis for income and expenditure, the software enables you to monitor the finances comprehensively.

Bank reconciliations are simple to do and at any time it is possible to access a screen showing the actual bank balance and the reconciled balance (which are not, of course, the same thing). If you want to be able to manage the finances of the practice, rather than just record the figures, then you will need a package such as this. Contact details are given at the end of this book for the Maclean McNicoll software. Your local computer dealer should have details of the Sage, Microsoft and Quicken packages.

In addition to a cashbook, most practice managers nowadays use spreadsheets – Excel or Lotus 123 – to help manage the accounts (*see* Question **67** on spreadsheets). Items-of-service claims can be monitored using a spreadsheet which will show up any variances month on month. Details of the petty cash can be kept in spreadsheet form as can information about cash paid into the practice in the form of private fees from patients, insurance companies and solicitors.

It is, of course, still possible to run the business using purely manual systems but the staff time saved using a computerized accounting system and the consequent reduced fees of the accountants can more than repay the initial outlay for appropriate software and any training required.

▲ Question 63: Payroll

Can you explain to me the advantages of doing the payroll on computer rather than the tried and tested manual system?

The main advantage has to be the accuracy and speed with which the computer can cope with a complex payrun. Doing the payroll manually can be very time consuming if you have a large number of staff, many of whom are working part time and perhaps doing regular overtime. It can also be fraught with difficulty if your calculations go awry. There are few sins considered as heinous as paying a member of staff less than they are entitled to, unless it is paying them too much and then having to ask for return of the overpayment.

If you use software produced specifically for general practice staff, such as the Ferguson payroll or GP staff wages system, you will find that all the idiosyncrasies, such as different levels of reimbursement and staff salaries deriving from separate budgets, including the fundholding management allowance, are taken into account when the calculations are done. For instance, with the Ferguson software you can allocate a set percentage of the ancillary staff salaries and NIC to the staff budget, but leave the cleaner's wages paid in full from the practice profits. You can also allocate the salaries of staff involved in fundholding to the management allowance or, if they have other duties within the practice, to a mixture of the management allowance and staff budget. The employer's NIC contribution for the GP registrar together with their total salary is automatically listed separately for reclaiming from the health authority. There is a facility to enter the registrar's car allowance and it can be taxed as appropriate. NHS pension deductions have been taken into account on the system and once you have input the relevant data regarding any overtime payments, maternity or sick pay, it is a simple matter to run the payroll.

Some practices continue to pay their staff weekly in cash which seems a very inefficient way of paying wages. The monthly salary paid directly into the staff's bank or building society accounts is quick and simple and a secure way of ensuring funds arrive in the bank accounts on the allotted day. If you use a computer to calculate the payrun for a staff of 25 or so, it should only take about half an hour to run on the computer, including printing off all the payslips, monthly statements of calculations and any giro cheques if you use the BACS system.

At the end of the financial year (which for the Inland Revenue will be 5 April) you will be required, like any other employer, to submit all the relevant calculations, including total salary paid and tax and NIC deducted for every member of staff employed by the practice during the financial year, whether partially reimbursed or not. A copy of the P60 will need to be given to each employee and sent to the Inland Revenue in duplicate. Having a computerized payroll will help you to produce all the required calculations for the Inland Revenue in a short space of time. Some systems will print the required information of yearly pay on special stationery that the tax office will accept at the end of the year and this will save you having to transcribe the details on to the Inland Revenue's special forms in triplicate.

▲ Question 64: Appointment system

We have recently installed an appointment system on our computer. Please tell me how we can make best use of this.

Computerized appointment systems are revolutionizing the way that practices can offer appointments. They have many advantages and the first that you will realize is that receptionists working at the front desk can now be available to welcome and deal with patients arriving in the surgery, rather than having to answer the telephone at the busiest times. Telephoned requests for appointments can be taken anywhere in the building where there is a computer terminal. At busy times such as first thing in the morning, therefore, several members of staff in other offices can be making appointments on the system while those at the desk deal with patients in person.

Once you have chosen and installed your appointment software, you will have to set up templates for the doctors' surgeries. This is the time to find out if any of the GPs wish to alter the length of consulting times for any of their surgeries. Those GPs who consistently run late might decide to see six or seven patients an hour rather than the usual eight and extend the surgery by half an hour or so in order to see the same number in total as the other doctors. Alternatively, one appointment slot could be blocked off every hour to allow for catching up or even provide time to drink a quick cup of coffee or to take patient telephone calls.

It is possible to set aside a certain proportion of slots so that they can only be booked by patients telephoning on the day with an urgent problem. It is also possible with most systems to make joint appointments so that the patient can see the nurse, followed by the GP or vice versa. Longer appointments can easily be made for patients who require extra time with their GP. Some practices ask the requesting patient whether they think they might require a double appointment for their particular problem. Surprisingly, research has shown that this is seldom abused and patients are often correct in their estimate of the time they will require. Often, giving the patient a longer time in which to discuss their problem in a little more depth can save them returning to see the GP again the following week.

From a management point of view, the auditing facility of computerized systems, such as the Frontdesk system produced by Informatica, is very useful. For instance, searches can be made for the number of patients seen in a given period by a particular clinician. This means that the partners can compare the number of patients each of them has seen during the past month or past quarter, which can be useful when they come to consider altering the surgery times. They can also monitor consultation times of the practice nurses and make any necessary changes to the time slots allowed.

The appointment history of a particular patient can be established at the press of a key, enabling you to see the frequency of their attendances at the practice or whether they have failed to turn up for booked appointments on several occasions. In this way, patients who persistently do not attend can be identified and appropriate action taken. GP workload can be audited and it should be possible to discover the percentage of patients seen by any one GP who are registered with another of the partners over a given period.

One facility which some systems have is for flashing urgent messages on to the screen in the GP's consulting room (*see* Question **65** on electronic messaging). This enables staff to alert a GP to an urgent matter during a consultation without the distraction of a telephone call, which is always an unwelcome interruption for GP and patient alike.

The only possible drawback with computerized appointment

systems is what would happen if there were a power cut or the computer system were to crash. As a precaution, one possible solution is to print off copies of the appointments for the day at the start of each morning and then these printed forms can be used as a basis to fill in the extras if necessary.

Many practices are reluctant to jettison their tried and tested appointments book. However, those who have transferred appointments to the computer wonder why they waited so long before making the transition. The benefits far outweigh any short-term disruption which is likely to be caused during the transition phase.

▲ Question 65: Electronic messaging

One business I know is able to flash messages on to the screens of all their users networked throughout the building. How can this be used in general practice?

Electronic messaging is a useful facility in any office situation but particularly in general practice where it allows members of staff to contact the doctor immediately, unobtrusively and silently without disrupting a consultation by telephoning. The message will be left on the screen for about three minutes and will remain stored for later recall. Thus, rather than offering an urgent appointment to all patients who telephone during the morning wishing to be seen immediately, the receptionist takes their telephone number and informs them that the doctor will call them back within ten minutes. The receptionist is freed from having to make decisions about the relative urgency of patients' stated problems and the system permits the doctor to deal with the problem over the telephone, if appropriate, and educate the patient at the same time about the actual urgency of his problem. For instance, some patients might be anxious to discuss the result of a particular test but it should not be necessary for them to make an appointment in order to do so. If results are kept on the computer, the GP could discuss any possible changes in medication or whatever briefly over the telephone, rather than call the patient in to see him.

It also helps if the practice is linked to the local laboratory, allowing results to be filed directly and automatically into the patient's computer record. Any GP who is still anxious about the medicolegal ramifications of keeping only computerized notes should be reassured by a recent test case in the courts which confirmed the legal validity of electronic medical records.

One possible problem with electronic messaging is that if the recipient of the message is not using their computer at the time the message is sent, the message may be overlooked. Another problem is that occasionally such messages can corrupt before the recipient has been able to make a note of the details. A way of checking that all messages have been acknowledged should be established. It might be a fail-safe system such as asking patients to call back in half an hour if the doctor has not yet contacted them.

▲ Question 66: Desktop publishing

We are wondering whether it is worthwhile producing our own headed paper and practice leaflets. Is this feasible using just the normal computer software?

There are potentially big savings to be made in producing your own stationery in-house. Which package you decide on will depend on how much you want to spend, which in turn will in all probability be related to how much you believe the practice can save by producing its own printed material. It will also depend on which particular software you already have on your system.

There is a software package for producing presentations called Powerpoint in the Microsoft Office Suite which enables the user to produce headed stationery, together with a logo or special image imported from Clipart, which might be sufficient for your needs.

Microsoft also produce a package called Publisher and their Word 97 software can be used to produce in-house printing as well. With any of these programs you should be able to produce leaflets in two or more columns and incorporate several colours into the design. The practice leaflet can be produced using this software but bear in mind that if you are planning to photocopy the print, you will need a colour photocopier if you opt for coloured text.

Desktop publishing allows you to experiment with producing printed material such as information leaflets on various health issues for handing out to patients by doctors or practice nurses. If you are interested in pursuing the idea you should consult a computer expert, explaining the equipment you have and what you require the software to do. You should find that you recoup the cost of any additional software you have to buy in a relatively short time and you certainly could have fun customizing and producing your own leaflets and headed paper.

▲ Question 67: Use of spreadsheets

I've never used spreadsheets before but understand that they can make managing the finances of a practice much simpler. I am going on a training course shortly in the use of Excel which I have on the PC in my office. What sort of spreadsheets should I be planning to set up?

Managers in general practice are increasingly using spreadsheets to monitor all aspects of the finances. For instance, you could register details of all staff salaries, including any increments due and the anticipated cost-of-living rise for the following year. From these figures you could extrapolate how much your staff budget would need to increase next year in order to cover 70% of ancillary staff salaries, together with 100% of employers' NIC. Any proposed bonuses could be added to the figures to see how they affect the overall budget.

You can use a spreadsheet to monitor items-of-service claims, noting the number of claims made (whether by Links or on forms sent) and the amount expected in payment for each claim. By creating a formula which multiplies the figure in one cell by the figure in another you can discover the anticipated total income for each category and compare this with the amount paid by the health authority at the end of the quarter. Any variances can then be investigated and a reason sought for the difference.

A spreadsheet on which you enter all electricity and gas quarterly payments is a useful way of identifying variances and keeping track of any unexpected rises in expenditure. The same could apply to telephone bills or any other cost that you wish to monitor. With the opportunity to use alternative suppliers for utilities and telephone nowadays, it is useful to do 'what if' calculations in order to help determine the least-cost option.

Producing a cashflow forecast is one of the most important tasks in managing the finances. It is a relatively simple task to set up a spreadsheet which will show the anticipated cashflow during the coming year. You should list anticipated income and expenditure and in the adjacent column should be entered the actual payments in and out as the figures become available. This will enable you to spot any variances between the estimated and actual figures and you can then seek reasons for such discrepancies. It is helpful to have a carry forward balance from month to month as this can be used to plan appropriate times for making expensive purchases or for transferring any surplus funds to a deposit account in anticipation of the biannual tax demands.

The facility with which you can recalculate figures simply is one of the main advantages of a spreadsheet. You can amend figures taking into account inflation or other anticipated factors which might affect outcomes and at the press of a key, see what difference the new figures will make. By altering just one figure you can gauge the knock-on effect this might have as the cells linked by formulae will all change correspondingly. For instance, you could see what impact on income a 5% increase, or decrease, in list size might have on the quarterly payments or what difference adjusting the payment of a specific standing order to quarterly from annually might make to the cashflow.

Many managers who have not yet used a spreadsheet find the prospect somewhat daunting. However, it really is relatively simple to learn the basics and as you become more proficient in using the software, you can create ever more ambitious spreadsheets to help you manage various aspects of the practice finances.

▲ Question 68: Word processing

The secretary in our practice is reluctant to jettison the old electronic typewriter and switch to word processing on the practice computer. What factors might help me to persuade her to make the change?

One of the myths about computers was that they were not suitable for real typists to use as their keyboards were not designed ergonomically in the same way that a typewriter keyboard is. This may have been the case at one time but it certainly is not so any more. Computer keyboards are light and well designed and can be used by someone typing at 100 wpm or with two fingers in a 'hunt and peck' manner.

There are many advantages to word processors, not least of which is the facility to rearrange the order of paragraphs or check and change spellings before printing out the result. Alternatively first drafts can be run off and amended simply on computer at a later date. For medical secretaries who have suffered from GPs dictating referral letters and then changing them substantially when they see the typed result, this can prove a real boon. If there is a prescribed limit to the number of words you can write in a given document, the word count facility is a very quick way of totting up the total number of words in the output so far.

The facility for mail merging, the process whereby data are drawn from the database on the system for incorporation into a standard document, should be a major factor in making such a decision. For instance, the patient's address or medical history can be accessed without having to input it via the keyboard individually. The same letter, such as a recall for cytology testing, can be written to women whose details can be extracted easily from the system. Any details can be changed as required prior to printing.

Copies of letters can be stored on the computer in a patient's medical record permanently. Hard copies can also be kept, of course, by the simple expedient of running off two copies of each document in order that one can be filed either in the patient's notes or in a chronological day file. Labels can be produced on sheets using a special template and this again can save time when you are doing a mass mailing. An envelope can be printed following production of a letter and this saves typing in the address twice.

The spell check facility and in-built thesaurus are very useful when composing reports. You might have to add medical terminology to the dictionary in the software but this is a small price to pay for being able to check a whole document in seconds for misspellings or typographical errors. It certainly cuts down the time required for proof reading lengthy documents.

I have known several typists who felt that the fact that they could type accurately at speed meant that they had no use for word processing. However, few reported any dissatisfaction with the new computer system once they had been encouraged to take the plunge and change. The initial training required to enable a competent typist to transfer to word processing is not great. If they know how to use a mouse and can access Windows, they are part of the way there. There are short courses available at most local colleges for beginners in word processing.

▲ Question 69: Computer crash

I am concerned about how we would cope if our computer were to crash. What contingency plans should we make?

The first and most obvious one is to ensure that you keep adequate back-ups of all data. In general practice it is usual to save data on to tape or disk at least once a day (often overnight). Whether you use disks or tapes you should rotate at least ten (*see* Question **73**), making sure that at least once a week a back-up tape is taken off the premises and stored at another location.

Some practices take the precaution of saving data on to a second hard disk. The only problem I see with this is that should the building be burnt down or the computers be stolen, you will still have lost everything. However, in the event of the main server crashing, it would be very convenient to be able to power up on the secondary machine with a minimum of delay and little loss of data so it is one option worth considering. (One GP with whom I discussed this paragraph remarked that this was definitely a 'belt and braces' approach.)

It is essential to set up a protocol so that staff know what they are expected to do in the event of a crisis such as a computer crash or break-in where the main server is stolen or damaged. The helpline numbers for your supplier should be readily available and details of how to obtain a replacement main server if it is required should be noted. How are you going to let patients know that there may be some problems with appointments immediately following the computer breakdown? Who else needs to be informed? How will you contact attached staff who might need the information contained on the computer?

Some appointment systems perform a back-up automatically throughout the day so appointments can be printed out from a PC if the server is stolen or crashes. However, if your system does not have this facility, you will need to decide how you are going to make new appointments if the staff had no time to print off forthcoming surgery appointments before the crash. Will the GPs hold open surgeries so that everyone can be seen in the hours (or days) immediately following the crash? Can and should the practice revert to using a manual system of making appointments until such time as the computer is reinstalled? And what about repeat prescriptions? Are there enough staff who know how to handwrite prescriptions until the system is back on-line?

You will no doubt be able to think of other problems of lack of access to the computer that will arise in your particular practice. With forethought and good forward planning, you should be able to limit the inevitable disruption.

▲ Question 70: Computer security

We have recently had a break-in at our practice when several of our PCs and printers were stolen. We have been told by our insurers that we need to improve our security before they will consider offering cover again on the equipment. Can you make any suggestions?

Burglars are increasingly targeting surgeries. Nowadays it is usually computers and other equipment such as mobile phones that they are after and not drugs. The fact is that, statistically, the premises are likely to be burgled more than once if thieves succeed in stealing computer equipment on the first occasion. Allowing a few weeks for you to replace the hardware, they will return once again and steal the new equipment. Sometimes they do not bother to remove the whole machine but just extract the essential and expensive microchips from inside the main server and any PCs. This process can be repeated each time you have had the opportunity to replace the stolen goods.

To minimize the chance of this happening to you, I would recommend that you seek the advice of a computer security expert who will illustrate the different systems for securing your equipment. If you make it sufficiently difficult for the thieves to obtain anything of value on their first visit, then they are less likely to return. Some of the different security systems include an entrapment device which is bolted to the floor and which encircles the main server, thus keeping it safe from removal by the opportunist burglar. It also ensures that the thief is unable to gain access to the computer by removing the back and stealing the chip.

Another system involves linking a strong cable through and around equipment which can then also be bolted to the floor. It is perhaps not resistant to a very determined burglar with heavy-duty cutters but should deter the all but the most determined thief. Any device that lengthens the time required to remove the equipment is useful as most burglars naturally want to be in and out in as short a time as possible to avoid detection.

Marking all the equipment with your postcode etched into the casing in a clearly visible place can be a deterrent to the thief since it will make resale of the stolen hardware more difficult, if not impossible. An alternative is to mark all portable computer equipment with a pen that shows up only under ultraviolet light. This will not deter the thief but may help in the recovery of marked property.

The security of the building itself may need to be looked at. By its very nature, a surgery has to be accessible to members of the public and this can obviously make security a particularly difficult problem. Some inner-city practices have had to resort to steel shutters, iron bars at the windows and panic buttons. However, this does little to prevent day-time opportunist thiefs. Further ideas for securing your building are given in answer to the question on the security of premises (see Question **29**).

▲ Question 71: Viruses

We are thinking of linking up to the Internet but I have heard that computer viruses are easily transmitted via the World Wide Web. How can we ensure that our system does not become infected?

The best way to ensure that your system does not take one of these viruses on board is to install a good antivirus program *before* you contemplate networking. Prevention is far simpler than cure in this instance. There are various antivirus 'toolkits' available, such as Dr Solomons (one of the most popular) and MacAfee, and you should check that the supplier of the one you choose provides regular updates to combat any new viruses that are circulating. Look in a recent computer magazine for details of antivirus programs which might be suitable and ask around among colleagues in other practices to find out what they do to prevent 'infection' by such bugs. There is a wide range of software available and the toolkits vary in price from a few pounds to several hundred.

▲ Question 72: Millennium time-bomb

We have been reading about the probability of computer crashes on the first day of the new century. How can we find out if all aspects of our system will be OK?

The threat of computer crashes at the start of the new century is called the Year 2000 Crisis or Y2K crisis for short. The software most likely to be affected are accounting systems (such as fundholding packages) and clinical systems where all entries are recorded by date and due dates are calculated with reference to these. However, other equipment such as BP monitors, autoclaves, telephone switchboards and central heating units which have a time chip in them may also be affected. To add to the confusion, the year 2000 is a leap year and many programers apparently did not take this into account when they wrote their programs. This means that some systems may not work at all on 29th February in the year 2000.

Health authorities circulated a document towards the end of 1997 stating that they would be responsible for any millennium changeover problems and it is assumed that this responsibility will also include paying the cost of making the required changes.

Suppliers are working hard to provide software which will help to avoid the predicted crash. However, it is likely that the proposed software will require at least a 486 computer in order to run. Upgrading 286 or 386 computers to this minimum required level is likely to cost thousands of pounds per practice. It is mainly the single-handed practices which are still using these slower computers and they are finding that health authority reimbursements towards the cost of upgrading cannot always be guaranteed. The Computer Services and Software Association has told the NHSE that 'A realistic estimate of the cost to upgrade GP systems would be £20-£30 million'. The sooner you ascertain the exact position regarding your own software and hardware and put in an application for possible reimbursement of new hardware, the better.

If you have Windows, a simple test to see if your system is likely to 'fall over' is to change the date and time settings in the 'set up' option to 31 December 1999 11.59 pm and then exit Windows and switch off the computer. Re-enter after a few minutes and check the date again. Microsoft expect 80% of computers will start up showing either 1980 or 1984 with this test. You must therefore upgrade immediately if your system is to manage the changeover to the new century without a hitch. There are various software packages to test software and hardware now available. Consult your supplier for details.

There is bound to be a last-minute panic with suppliers being inundated with calls as the end of 1999 approaches. By then it will be too late to do anything. It is important that you do not delay and make the necessary changes now in good time for the change-over. Do not forget to check all other equipment that might have a chip installed.

▲ Question 73: Computer back-ups

I understand that we should back up our computer data in case we have a computer crash. Can you tell me how frequently this should be done and when?

It is advisable to back up the data on your clinical system every working day. Most systems have a facility to set the back-up going automatically during the night so that users are not required to log out during office hours. If you have a tape streamer you can usually obtain a tape of sufficient size to enable all your data to be backed up onto one tape. These tapes should be rotated and you will require ten for an effective back-up system. Five will be used for the daily back-ups and one of these should be taken out of the building and kept for a week. The other four can then be reused the following week together with a new one, which will also need to be taken out of the building for safe deposit elsewhere. At the end of the month you will need to take a monthly back-up and when this tape has been verified, the other previous back-ups can then be reused in rotation once again. This system ensures that you always have several recent back-up copies of data should the system crash or in the event of total destruction of the hard disk at the practice through fire or burglary.

There is no point doing back-ups unless you have verified the tape or disk. It is important to check the anticipated life of the tape with the supplier. If it is 50 applications, then rotating the tape weekly would mean that it should be replaced annually. If the tape is used beyond its expected life capacity, then the data will not back up accurately and the tape will be useless if and when you come to restore the data.

Alternatively, some practices choose to have a separate hard disk onto which data are backed up. This can pose problems if there is a fire and both hard disks are kept in the same building. I cannot stress too strongly that it is essential to keep an up-to-date-back up tape at another location at all times in case of fire or theft. Practices who have failed to do this and have had their hardware containing years of data stolen or destroyed have had to start from scratch which is a daunting prospect. It is not just the expense of replacing the system but also the time factor involved in staff having to replace as much of the patient data as possible from other sources.

Further reading

Baker R and Presley P (1990) *The Practice Audit Plan: a handbook of medical audit*. RCGP Severn Faculty. Bristol.

DoH (1997) *The New NHS: modern – dependable*, HMSO, London.

Ellis N (1994) *Making Sense of General Practice*. Radcliffe Medical Press, Oxford.

Ellis N (ed) (1997) *General Practitioner's Handbook*. Radcliffe Medical Press, Oxford.

Ellis N and Chisholm J (1997) *Making Sense of the Red Book*. Radcliffe Medical Press, Oxford.

Huntington J (1995) *Managing the Practice: whose business?* Radcliffe Medical Press, Oxford.

Irvine D (1990) *Managing for Quality in General Practice*. King's Fund, London.

Irvine D and Irvine S (eds) (1997) *Making Sense of Audit* (2nd ed). Radcliffe Medical Press, Oxford.

Irvine D and Irvine S (1996) *The Practice of Quality*. Radcliffe Medical Press, Oxford.

Sheldon MG (1985) *Trends in GP Computing*. Royal College of General Practitioners, London.

Useful addresses

Association of Managers in General Practice (AMGP)
Suite 308
The Foundry
156 Blackfriars Road
London SE1 8EN
Tel: 0171 721 7080

Association of Medical Secretaries, Practice Managers, Administrators and Receptionists (AMSPAR)
Tavistock House North
Tavistock Square
London WC1H 9LN
Tel: 0171 387 6005

British Medical Association
BMA House
Tavistock Square
London WC1H 9JP
Tel: 0171 387 4499

Croner Publications Ltd
Croner House
London Road
Kingston upon Thames
Surrey KT2 6SR
Tel: 0181 547 3333
Fax: 0181 547 2637

Data Protection Agency
Wycliffe House
Water Lane
Wilmslow
Cheshire SK9 5AF
Tel: 01625 545700
Fax: 01625 524510

Health and Safety Executive
Information Centre
Broad Lane
Sheffield S3 7HQ
Tel: 0541 545500

Health and Safety Executive Books
P O Box 1999
Sudbury
Suffolk CO10 6FS
Tel: 01787 881165
Fax: 01787 313995

Practice Manager
George Warman Publications
Unit 2, Riverview Business Park
Walnut Tree Close
Guildford
Surrey GU1 4UX
Tel: 01483 304944

Royal College of General Practitioners
14 Princes Gate
Hyde Park
London SW7 1PU
Tel: 0171 581 3232
Fax: 0171 225 3046

Computer experts specializing in general practice computing needs

PCTI Solutions Ltd (Professional Computer Training and Installation)
Churchill House
Mill Hill Road
Pontefract
W Yorkshire WF8 4HY
Tel: 01977 690977
Fax: 01977 690966

Visual Productions (computerized Red Book)
41 Grove Avenue
Coombe Dingle
Bristol BS9 2RP
0117 907 7501

Computer software suppliers

Ferguson GP Software (payroll)
5 Craignethan Road
Glasgow G46 6SQ
Helpline: 0831 387 068 (Mon and Wed pm)
Fax: 0141 616 0691

GP staff wages system
Dr A Crawshaw
Hill Top House
Mevagissey
Cornwall PL26 6RY
Tel: 01726 843595

Maclean McNicoll Software
Holmfield
Duntocher Road
Clydebank G81 3LN
Ansafone/fax: 0141 952 9707

Microsoft Ltd (Microsoft Money)
Microsoft Campus
Thames Valley Park
Reading RG6 1WG
Tel: 0345 002000

Quicken
Intuit Service Centre
P O Box 139
Chertsey
Surrey KT16 9FE
Tel: 0800 585058
Fax: 01932 578522

Index